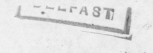

Essential Medicines

Essential Medicine

J. L. Burton B.Sc., M.D., F.R.C.P.

Consultant Senior Lecturer in Dermatology,
Bristol Royal Infirmary

CHURCHILL LIVINGSTONE
EDINBURGH LONDON MELBOURNE AND NEW YORK 1981

CHURCHILL LIVINGSTONE
Medical Division of Longman Group Limited

Distributed in the United States of America by Churchill
Livingstone Inc., 19 West 44th Street, New York, N.Y.
10036, and by associated companies, branches and
representatives throughout the world.

First published 1981

A version of this book was published in 1976 under the title
Aids to Medicine for Nurses.

ISBN 0 443 02438 3

British Library Cataloguing in Publication Data
Burton J. L.
Essential medicine.
  1. Medicine   2. Nursing
  I. Title
  610'.24613   RT65

Printed in Hong Kong by
Sheck Wah Tong Printing Press Ltd

Preface

Nurses and medical students are faced with a daunting task when they first begin their training on a medical ward. The sheer volume of knowledge which has to be assimilated means that often they cannot see 'the wood for the trees'. This little book aims to provide a simple and succinct account of general medicine which can be read easily and quickly and then used as a basis for further study of the larger and more comprehensive textbooks.

I hope that nurses will find it useful throughout their training, and also for rapid revision of essential facts just before examinations. Medical students should find it helpful as an introductory text on their first medical 'firm', and para-medical students such as physiotherapists and radiographers may also find it useful.

Each chapter gives a brief review of the important anatomy and physiology of a particular system, followed by the causes, clinical features, complications and treatment of the common diseases which occur in that system. There are also chapters on medical terminology and on the uses of common drugs.

This book was originally published as *Aids to Medicine for Nurses* but with the change in format the book has been re-titled *Essential Medicine*. It has been completely updated, and enlarged by the addition of several new chapters and more than 50 new diagrams.

Once again I should like to thank my nursing colleagues in the School of Nursing in the Bristol Health District who have been most helpful and have made a number of very valuable suggestions.

1981   J.L.B.

Contents

1 Medical terminology

Disease

Broadly speaking, any alteration of the structure or function of the organs or tissues of the body may be called a disease.

Symptoms

These are what the patient complains of, e.g. pain or tiredness.
They are obtained by taking a history from the patient.

Signs

These are the physical abnormalities found on examining the patient. The physical examination by a physician usually proceeds in the following stages:

1. Inspection i.e. looking
2. Palpation i.e. feeling with the hands or fingers
3. Percussion i.e. one finger is placed firmly on the part to be tested and is then tapped with the finger-tip of the opposite hand to detect whether the tissue has the normal resonance. The resonance may be increased by excessive gas or decreased by excessive fluid
4. Auscultation i.e. listening with a stethoscope

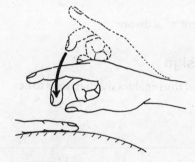

Figure 1.1
Percussion

Syndrome

A set of symptoms and signs which characterize a particular disease.

Diagnosis

The recognition of a particular disease from its symptoms, signs and any special tests.

Differential diagnosis

A list of similar diseases from one of which the patient may be suffering.

Prognosis

The prediction of the duration and outcome of a disease and its likely response to treatment.

Complications

These are developments of the original disease which do not occur in every patient, but which adversely affect the prognosis.

Sequelae

These are the long-term results which follow from a particular disease or its treatment.

Prophylaxis

The prevention of disease.

Aetiology

The various factors involved in the causation of a disease.

Pathogenesis

The mode of production or development of a disease.

Pathognomonic symptom or sign

One which occurs in only one disease, and thus enables the diagnosis to be made.

Types of disease

Diseases may be classified in many ways, but most can be fitted into one or more of the following categories:

1. *Congenital*
   This dates from birth.
   A congenital disease may be hereditary (i.e. inherited due to a genetic disorder), or it may be due to damage to the fetus caused by drugs or infection which can cross the placenta. Diseases which tend to run in the family are said to be *familial,* but they may not be congenital (e.g. hay fever).

2. *Physical damage* (trauma)
   This includes accidental or intentional violence, surgical operations, excessive heat, cold, radiation or corrosive chemicals which cause tissue damage.

3. *Mechanical defects*
   These include various factors which obstruct tubes or vessels e.g. blood clot in a vein, adhesions of the bowel.

4. *Infection or infestation*
   Various living organisms may cause disease by invading the patient. These include (in ascending order of size):

(i) *Viruses* e.g. Varicella (chicken-pox) and measles
(ii) *Bacteria*
    a. Cocci — round organisms e.g. Staphylococci and Streptococci
    b. Bacilli — rod-shaped organisms e.g. Mycobacterium tuberculosis
    c. Treponemes — corkscrew-shaped organisms e.g. Treponema pallidum (Syphilis)
(iii) *Protozoa* e.g. malaria and amoebic dysentery
(iv) *Fungi* e.g. dermatophytes and yeasts
(v) *Animal parasites* e.g. mites, worms, lice

5. *Neoplasia* (new growths)

Strictly speaking, a tumour is any kind of abnormal swelling, but most tumours are due to neoplasia. A neoplasm is a new growth of cells which is uncontrolled and unnecessary for the function of the body.

A *benign* neoplasm has the following features:
(i) Its cells resemble those of the tissue from which they arise
(ii) It is usually slow-growing
(iii) It usually has a capsule
(iv) It does not invade normal surrounding tissue
(v) It does not spread to distant parts of the body

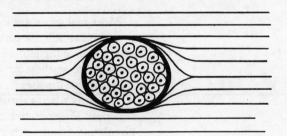

Figure 1.2
Benign tumour. Pressure effects only

Benign tumours usually take their name from their tissue of origin, and they may arise from most tissues:
e.g. *Fibroma* from fibrous tissue
    Lipoma from fat
    Neuroma from nerve
    Angioma from a vessel
    Osteoma from bone

A *malignant* neoplasm has the following features:
(i) Its cells may not resemble the cells of the tissue from which they arise. These tumours are said to be anaplastic and they have a poor prognosis
(ii) Its cells divide rapidly, often with abnormal nuclei
(iii) It has no capsule
(iv) It usually invades the underlying tissues
(v) It tends to spread (metastasize) to distant parts of the body, either via the blood-stream (haematogenous dissemination) or via the lymphatic vessels (lymphatic dissemination)

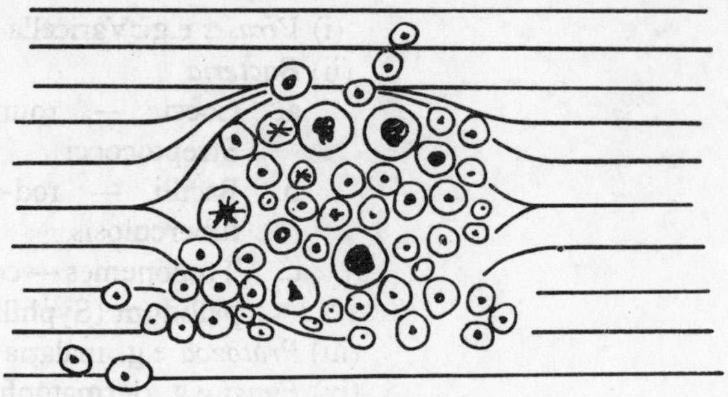

Figure 1.3
Malignant tumour. Pressure effects
and invasion

Malignant tumours are of several types:

1. *Carcinoma* (cancer) originates from a 'lining tissue' (epithelium) such as skin, bronchus or intestinal epithelium. Some cancers are often fatal (e.g. gastric cancer) and others are rarely fatal if treated early (e.g. basal cell cancer of skin)
2. *Sarcoma* originates from a deeper tissue (mesoderm) such as muscle or bone. Sarcoma usually has a poor prognosis
3. *Lymphoma* originates in the reticulo-endothelial cells of the lymphoid tissue, and there are varying degrees of malignancy
4. *Leukaemia* originates in the 'stem cells' which divide to produce white cells (leucocytes)

Most malignant tumours have a poor prognosis but some benign tumours can kill the patient because of their huge size (e.g. ovarian), and some malignant tumours (e.g. basal cell skin cancer) do not metastasize so they can be completely cured.

6. *Degenerative disease*
This occurs when a tissue ages or 'wears out', so that it loses its normal function. Degenerative changes in the heart and blood vessels lead to circulatory failure. An inadequate blood supply to an organ is called *ischaemia*. This usually produces *anoxia* (lack of oxygen) in the tissue, and if the tissue becomes *necrotic* (dies) as a result, this is called *infarction*.

7. *Metabolic disease*
The innumerable biochemical reactions which occur in the body are vital for health, and derangement of this normal metabolism (e.g. by an enzyme deficiency) can cause serious disease.

The endocrine glands secrete hormones which regulate metabolic activity, and over-activity or underactivity of an endocrine gland usually causes disease.

The various components of the diet (fat, carbohydrate, protein, mineral salts, vitamins and water) are also essential for normal metabolism, and excess or deficiency of one or more of these dietary components can cause disease.

8. *Immunological disease*
The body has a number of complex defence mechanisms which help it to prevent infections, but if infection does occur, these immune mechanisms play an important role in producing the changes of inflammation (redness, heat, swelling and tenderness).

There are many ways in which these immunological mechanisms can become deranged and cause disease. Abnormal antibodies may attack the body's own tissue, as in thyroiditis due to anti-thyroid antibodies, or they may cause allergy to an external substance, as in hay-fever, due to pollen allergy. An *allergen* is a substance which is harmless to normal people, but which provokes an abnormal immunological reaction in a person who is sensitized to it. In hay-fever, the allergen is pollen from a particular plant.

More complex immunological abnormalities are involved in the so-called 'collagen-vascular' diseases such as rheumatoid arthritis and systemic lupus erythematosus.

9. *Disease due to drugs or poisons*

As more and more powerful drugs become available to doctors, *side-effects* are becoming increasingly important. Some side-effects are *dose-related* i.e. they would affect everyone in the same way if a big enough dose were given, and others are *idiosyncratic* i.e. they adversely affect only a few individuals, and a large dose is not required for the side-effect to be produced. Sometimes a drug acts as an allergen and provokes an immunological disorder.

The effect of poisons is usually dose-related, and any drug or chemical, even common salt, is poisonous to man if taken in sufficient quantity.

2 Cardiovascular system

The heart is a muscle pump whose function is to perfuse the tissues with blood by contracting rhythmically. In a resting adult the heart expels about 5 litres of blood each minute (*cardiac output*).

The *pericardium* is a two-layered sac which encloses the heart.

The *myocardium* is the heart muscle.

The *endocardium* lines the 4 heart chambers and covers the 4 heart valves.

The 4 chambers are:
1. The R. and L. atria
2. The R. and L. ventricles

The 4 valves are:
1. The aortic and pulmonary valves
2. The mitral and tricuspid valves

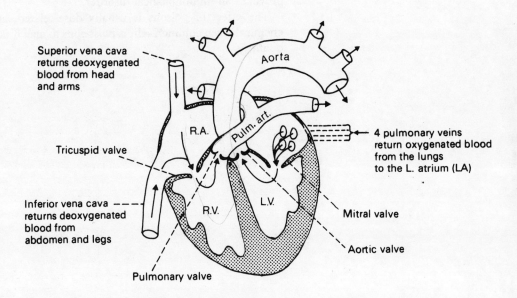

Superior vena cava returns deoxygenated blood from head and arms

Aorta

R.A.

Pulm. art.

4 pulmonary veins return oxygenated blood from the lungs to the L. atrium (LA)

Tricuspid valve

Inferior vena cava returns deoxygenated blood from abdomen and legs

R.V.

L.V.

Mitral valve

Aortic valve

Pulmonary valve

Figure 2.1

Pulmonary and systemic circulation

The heart acts like two separate pumps which act side by side.

The right pump (RA and RV) is responsible for pumping blood to and through the lungs. This is the pulmonary circulation, which drains into the LA.

The left pump (LA and LV) pumps blood throughout the rest of the body. This is the systemic circulation, which drains into the RA.

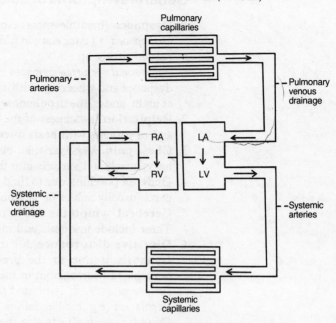

PULMONARY CIRCULATION (RV TO LA)

Pulmonary
capillaries

Pulmonary
arteries

Pulmonary
venous
drainage

RA   LA

RV   LV

Systemic
venous
drainage

Systemic
arteries

Systemic
capillaries

SYSTEMIC CIRCULATION (LV TO RA)

Figure 2.2
The circulation of blood. Note that
the heart acts as two separate
pumps

The cardiac cycle

Atrial contraction (*atrial systole*) squeezes blood into the ventricles while
they are relaxed (*ventricular diastole*). The ventricles then contract
(*ventricular systole*) to expel blood into the aorta and R. and L. pulmonary
arteries while the atria relax (*atrial diastole*) and refill with blood from the
superior and inferior venae cavae and pulmonary veins.

This regular sequence of contraction is maintained by electrical
impulses which originate from the *sino-atrial node (pacemaker)* in the R.
atrium. Each impulse spreads in all directions over both atria, and after a
short delay at the *atrioventricular node* it travels rapidly down the
specialized conducting tissue (*atrioventricular bundle*) in the
interventricular septum to stimulate both ventricles. After each impulse
the conducting tissue requires a short rest period (*refractory period*)
before another impulse can pass.

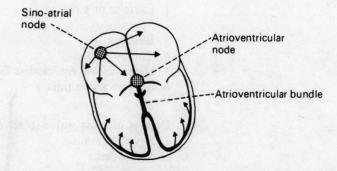

Sino-atrial
node

Atrioventricular
node

Atrioventricular bundle

Figure 2.3

General symptoms of heart disease

1. **Dyspnoea** (breathlessness) especially on exertion
   Orthopnoea is a later stage in which breathlessness forces the patient to remain sitting up
   Paroxysmal nocturnal dyspnoea is characterized by the sudden onset of dyspnoea and wheezing, with a sense of suffocation. It usually occurs at night, and is due to pulmonary congestion with the patient lying flat
2. **Palpitation** (awareness of the heart beat) occurs in normal subjects and in patients with heart disease
3. **Chest pain.** Very variable, but often precipitated by exertion or a heavy meal, and spreads into the neck or arms
4. **Oedema** (swelling due to fluid accumulation) of the most dependent parts (usually ankles or sacrum)
5. **Cerebral symptoms** due to impaired oxygenation of the brain. These include insomnia and memory loss
6. **Digestive disturbance** due to gastrointestinal congestion
7. **Cyanosis** is due to the presence of an excess of inadequately oxygenated haemoglobin in the blood
   Peripheral cyanosis is limited to the extremities and is due to poor circulation (e.g. cardiac failure, or vasoconstriction due to cold)
   Central cyanosis affects also the lips and tongue
   Causes of central cyanosis:
   1. Impaired oxygenation of blood in lungs
   2. Congenital heart disease with a R. to L. 'shunt' of blood (e.g. Fallot's tetralogy)

The arterial pulse

Observe	1. Rate
	2. Rhythm
	3. Character

1. RATE

Normal:	Resting adult	60–85 beats/min
	Resting child	80–100 beats/min
	Newborn infant	100–130 beats/min

Causes of rapid pulse (tachycardia)
1. Exercise or emotion
2. Fever
3. Bleeding
4. Thyrotoxicosis
5. Heart disease e.g. cardiac failure
6. Cardiac arrhythmia

Causes of slow pulse (bradycardia)
1. Physical training
2. Myxoedema

3. Raised intra-cranial pressure
4. Drugs e.g. digitalis
5. Heart block

Pulse deficit. If some ventricular contractions fail to produce a radial pulse beat the *apex rate* (felt or heard at the heart apex) will exceed the rate at the wrist. This is called a 'pulse deficit' and it implies that the heart is not contracting efficiently so that some beats are wasted. A pulse deficit is often an early sign of digoxin overdosage.

Causes of a pulse deficit
1. Extrasystoles
2. Atrial fibrillation

2. RHYTHM

Common causes of an irregular pulse
1. Sinus arrhythmia
2. Extrasystoles
3. Atrial fibrillation

1. Sinus arrhythmia
A physiological increase in pulse rate during inspiration. Common in children and during convalescence.

2. Extrasystole (ectopic beat)

Figure 2.4
Pulse waves showing extrasystole.
Note the compensatory pause after
the early beat

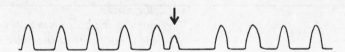

An extrasystole is a premature beat due to a cardiac impulse arising at an abnormal (ectopic) site in the heart. The pulse beat felt at the wrist is usually weak. This is followed by a *compensatory pause* and the next beat is unusually forceful. Extrasystoles are common and may not be dangerous.

Causes of extrasystoles
 (i) Fatigue
 (ii) Excessive smoking or ingestion of alcohol or coffee
(iii) Heart disease e.g. mitral stenosis or myocardial ischaemia
(iv) Drugs e.g. digitalis
 (v) Thyrotoxicosis

3. Atrial fibrillation
Very rapid uncoordinated contractions of muscle bundles occur all over the atria, and the ventricles are stimulated rapidly and irregularly. The pulse rate is about 100–180 beats/min unless controlled by digitalis.

Causes of atrial fibrillation
  (i) Rheumatic heart disease (e.g. mitral stenosis)
 (ii) Myocardial ischaemia
(iii) Thyrotoxicosis

3. CHARACTER (Quality)

(i) *Volume*
A full 'bounding' pulse may be due to a hyperdynamic circulation e.g. fever, pregnancy, thyrotoxicosis.

A weak pulse may be due to dehydration, blood loss, myocardial infarction or 'shock'.

Pulsus alternans occurs when the volume of the pulse is alternately large and small in a regular sequence. It is a sign of severe heart failure.

Pulsus alternans may be observed by palpation of the radial pulse, or it may be observed while taking the blood pressure.

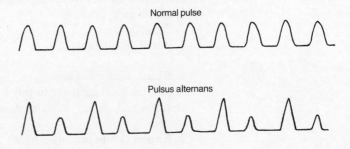

Normal pulse

Pulsus alternans

Figure 2.5

(ii) *Pulse wave*
Variations in the pulse wave may be helpful in diagnosis.

In aortic *incompetence* the pulse beat has a 'slapping' quality (*collapsing pulse*).

In aortic *stenosis* the pulse beat is sustained (*plateau pulse*).

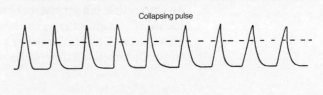

Collapsing pulse

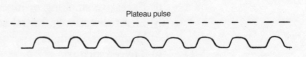

Plateau pulse

Figure 2.6

(iii) *State of the artery*
Normal arteries are soft and elastic.
Arteriosclerotic arteries are hard and rigid.

Cardiac arrhythmias

1. Extrasystoles (p. 9)

2. Atrial fibrillation (p. 9)

3. Atrial flutter

An uncommon arrhythmia due to heart disease. The pulse rate is rapid and regular but may vary due to changes in the degree of heart block (q.v.).

4. Paroxysmal tachycardia

Rapid heart-beats, often of sudden onset, due to regular discharge of impulses from an ectopic focus in the atria, atrioventricular node or ventricles. The attacks cause palpitations and usually stop suddenly after a few seconds, minutes or days.

Heart block

This refers to impairment of the conduction of the impulses through the AV node and the atrio-ventricular bundle. Mild degrees may be seen only on an electrocardiogram, but in more severe degrees there is bradycardia (about 36 beats/min) with the atria and ventricles contracting independently of each other.

Stokes-Adams attacks are periods of unconsciousness from cerebral anoxia due to transient cardiac arrest as a result of unstable heart block. The patient is very pale during the attack but becomes flushed as consciousness returns.

Jugular venous pulse (J.V.P.)

The pressure in the jugular veins can be estimated by inspecting the neck in the recumbent patient with the head and shoulders raised 30° from the horizontal. The pressure is increased in heart failure and in obstruction of the superior vena cava.

Blood pressure

In taking the blood-pressure (BP) the observer applies the armband of the sphygmomanometer firmly and evenly around the arm about two inches above the elbow. The arm band is then blown up until the brachial artery is occluded and at this point the radial pulse disappears. The stethoscope is then placed over the brachial artery at the elbow and the observer auscultates as the pressure is released.

A soft puffing noise is heard at and below systolic pressure, and as the diastolic pressure is approached the sound gradually becomes much sharper, and then suddenly changes to a much softer sound which fades away. Strictly speaking the point of transition from the loud knocking sound to the soft blowing sound is the diastolic pressure, but often the distinction is not clear.

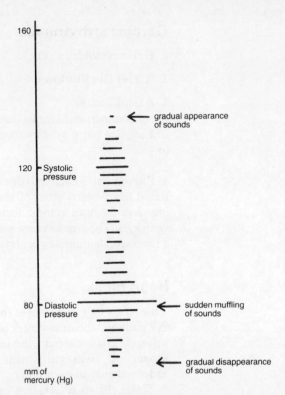

Figure 2.7
Blood pressure

In some patients with hypertension the sounds may disappear midway between systolic and diastolic pressure, and so the systolic pressure should first be checked by palpation of the radial pulse at the wrist.

The BP should be measured with the patient resting and relaxed. It rises with age but normal values in adults are:

Systolic = 100 to 140 mm Hg

Diastolic = 60 to 90 mm Hg

Pulse pressure (systolic minus diastolic) = 30 to 60 mm Hg. Old people with arteriosclerosis often have a raised systolic pressure and a normal diastolic pressure. This is of little significance, but increased diastolic pressure is always important.

HYPOTENSION

Low systolic BP

Causes
1. Vasovagal attack ('fainting')
2. Systemic infections e.g. 'flu', enteric fever
3. Myocardial infarction
4. Dehydration or bleeding
5. Hypoadrenalism

Symptoms of hypotension
1. Weakness or faintness, especially on standing
2. Giddiness, mental confusion or 'blacking-out' of vision

Complications of hypotension

Prolonged and severe hypotension may cause permanent damage to the brain or kidneys.

Treatment of hypotension

In severe hypotension the patient should be nursed flat, with the legs elevated, and the underlying cause should be treated.

In some types of acute hypotension (e.g. due to bleeding) rapid transfusion with plasma or blood may be required.

SYSTEMIC HYPERTENSION
BP more than 150/90

Causes
1. Essential hypertension (cause unknown)
2. Secondary
   (i) Renal disease e.g. nephritis or renal ischaemia
   (ii) Rarely coarctation of aorta, phaeochromocytoma, Cushing's disease etc.

Malignant hypertension is severe hypertension characterized by a diastolic pressure over 140 mm Hg, retinal changes (papilloedema and haemorrhages) and progressive renal failure

Symptoms of hypertension
1. May be no symptoms
2. 'Fullness' in the head, throbbing headache, giddiness or palpitations

Complications of hypertension
1. Left ventricular failure
2. Arterial degeneration (atheroma)
3. Retinopathy (retinal bleeding, exudate or papilloedema)
4. Albuminuria and renal failure
5. Cerebral thrombosis or haemorrhage (p. 75)

Treatment of hypertension
1. Weight reduction, avoidance of stress and strain, stopping smoking
2. Drugs — for mild hypertension (diastolic 90 to 110 mm Hg) a sedative or a regular diuretic such as *chlorothiazide* may be sufficient. Drugs for moderate or severe hypertension include *propranolol*, *methyldopa* and *bethanidine*. Treatment is for life, and regular BP checks are required.

PULMONARY HYPERTENSION

An increased pressure in the pulmonary circulation may occur in several ways:

1. Failure of the left side of the heart may cause increased back-pressure in the lungs, secondary to the raised pressure in the left atrium.
2. Blood may be shunted from the left side of the heart to the right side through a hole in the atrial or ventricular septa (p. 16), and therefore the pulmonary circulation becomes overloaded.

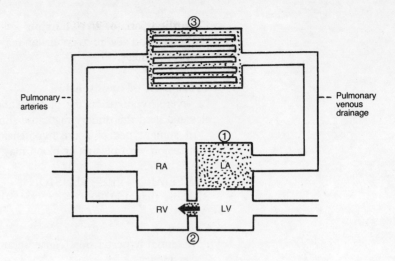

Figure 2.8
Causes of pulmonary hypertension

① Secondary to increased pressure in L. atrium

② Abnormal shunt from L. side to R. side of heart

③ Pulmonary disease

3. Constriction or obstruction of the small vessels in the lungs may occur in a variety of respiratory diseases e.g. bronchitis or pulmonary emboli (p. 24), etc.

HEART SOUNDS AND MURMURS

The heart sounds heard through a stethoscope occur in pairs. The first sound ('Lub') is due to simultaneous closure of the mitral and triscuspid valves, and the second sound ('Dup') is due to closure of the aortic and pulmonary valves. Ventricular systole occurs between these two sounds, and ventricular diastole occurs in the interval between each pair of sounds.

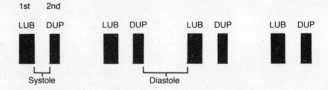

Figure 2.9

The first sound is normally louder than the second sound, and the diastolic interval is longer than the systolic interval.

Sounds due to an abnormal blood flow are called *murmurs* or *bruits*.

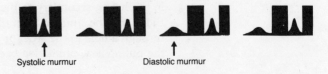

Figure 2.10

Murmurs may occur either in systole or diastole. They may indicate a structural abnormality in the heart or great vessels, but many murmurs, especially in children, are 'innocent' i.e. they have no pathological significance.

Valvular disease

CAUSES

1. Congenital

2. Rheumatic heart disease (p. 17)

3. Infective endocarditis (p. 18)

4. Syphilis (p. 18)

CONGENITAL HEART DISEASE

Classified into 2 groups, cyanotic and acyanotic according to whether the patient is cyanosed or not.

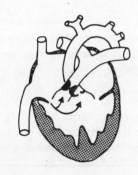

Figure 2.11

1. Cyanotic
Fallot's tetralogy, the commonest example, consists of:

1. Pulmonary stenosis
2. Ventricular septal defect
3. Over-riding aorta, which lies over both ventricles
4. R. ventricular hypertrophy

Clinical features of Fallot's tetralogy:
1. Cyanosis and polycythaemia
2. Dyspnoea on exertion (relieved by squatting)
3. Clubbing of fingers
4. Impaired growth
5. Systolic heart murmur

2. Acyanotic (i.e. without cyanosis)

Coarctation of the aorta
Narrowing of the aorta, usually just below the L subclavian artery. The BP is usually raised in the head and arms, but the femoral pulses are delayed and diminished. The prognosis is variable.

Treatment
Surgical excision of the narrowed portion.

Persistent ductus arteriosus
In an adult the pressure in the aorta is higher than in the pulmonary artery, but in the fetus the reverse is true. Before birth the lungs are not needed, and so most of the blood by-passes the lungs by a duct from the

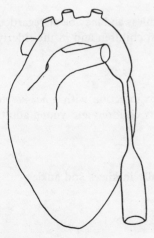

Figure 2.12
Coarctation of the aorta

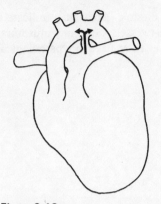

Figure 2.13
Ductus arteriosus in a fetus. Blood flows from pulmonary artery to aorta

pulmonary artery to the artery. This duct normally closes at birth, but if it remains patent the direction of blood flow reverses and the pulmonary circulation becomes overloaded. These patients may develop cardiac failure or subacute bacterial endocarditis (p. 18).

Treatment
Infusion of prostaglandin will sometimes close the duct, but if this fails, it is ligated surgically.

Pulmonary stenosis (narrowing of the pulmonary valve)
Mild cases may have no symptoms but severe cases develop cardiac failure before middle life.

SEPTAL DEFECTS
A failure of normal development in the fetus may produce a congenital hole in the septum between the two atria, or in the septum between the two ventricles.

Atrial septal defect
Blood from the L. atrium passes through the hole into the R. atrium and thus re-enters the pulmonary circulation. There may be few symptoms until middle age, when cardiac failure develops.

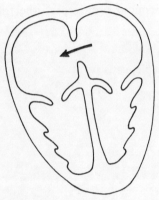

Figure 2.14
Atrial septal defect. Blood flows from L. atrium to R. atrium

Ventricular septal defect
A small defect will produce a murmur without symptoms, but a large defect will allow so much blood to enter the R. ventricle from the L. ventricle that the pulmonary circulation becomes overloaded and pulmonary hypertension develops.

Treatment
In some cases none is required, but if necessary the defect can be closed surgically.

'Innocent' murmurs
The majority of systolic murmurs are harmless and may be disregarded. These 'innocent' murmurs are common in children and in the elderly.

RHEUMATIC FEVER
Aetiology. Probably an allergic reaction to infection with a *haemolytic Streptococcus* (usually tonsillitis). It affects children and young adults, but is now uncommon in Britain.

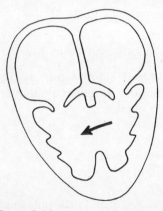

Figure 2.15
Ventricular septal defect. Blood flows from L. ventricle to R. ventricle

Clinical features
1. Fever and 'flitting' joint pains, especially in knees and ankles
2. Cardiac involvement
   (i) Tachycardia
   (ii) Cardiac murmurs
   (iii) Cardiac enlargement or failure
   (iv) Pericarditis

3. Rash or subcutaneous nodules

Treatment
1. Rest, with support for the joints and a high fluid intake
2. Salicylates such as aspirin in high dosage
   Steroid therapy is sometimes used for carditis
3. Penicillin may be used to eradicate the Streptococcus and long-term penicillin prevents further attacks

Complete rest must be enforced for many weeks, until all signs of active disease have gone and the plasma viscosity or ESR is normal.

Rheumatic chorea
This is a similar allergic process affecting the brain. Affected children become restless and fidgety, with involuntary movements and grimaces. The disease lasts about 2 months, but some cases develop rheumatic heart disease.

RHEUMATIC HEART DISEASE
Rheumatic fever causes endocarditis with small 'vegetations' (fibrin, platelets and leucocytes) on the valves. These are replaced by fibrous scar tissue which gradually contracts and deforms the valve so it either becomes narrowed (*stenosis*) or fails to close properly (*incompetence*). There is usually a latent period of 15–20 years before symptoms such as dyspnoea appear. The mitral and aortic valves are most commonly affected.

Mitral stenosis
Mitral stenosis obstructs the flow from L. atrium to L. ventricle and this causes a rise in pressure in the L. atrium. At first the heart compensates by enlargement of the atrium and hypertrophy of its walls, but later the pressure in the pulmonary circulation rises. The resulting pulmonary congestion causes dyspnoea and the patient may develop attacks of acute pulmonary oedema. Eventually R. ventricular failure occurs.

Closed   Open

Normal mitral valve

Figure 2.16

Clinical features
1. Pulmonary congestion
   (i) Progressive exertional dyspnoea
   (ii) Orthopnoea (dyspnoea when lying flat)
   (iii) Paroxysmal nocturnal dyspnoea ('cardiac asthma')
   (iv) Cough and haemoptysis
2. Loud first heart sound with a soft diastolic murmur
3. Often a thin face with purple cheeks ('malar flush')

Complications
1. Atrial fibrillation
2. Acute pulmonary oedema
3. R. ventricular failure
4. Thrombus in L. atrium and systemic emboli (e.g. cerebral)
5. Subacute bacterial endocarditis (p. 18)
6. Recurrent bronchitis

Treatment
1. Treatment of cardiac failure (p. 19)
2. Mitral valvotomy or valve replacement

Mitral incompetence
This may be due to rheumatic heart disease or it may be secondary to L. ventricular failure and dilatation. There is a loud systolic murmur at the apex which is caused by blood regurgitating from the left ventricle into the left atrium.

Treatment
1. Treatment of cardiac failure
2. In severe cases, valve replacement may be needed

Aortic stenosis
This causes a harsh systolic murmur over the aorta but there may be few symptoms for many years. Eventually L. ventricular failure, angina or syncope ('black-outs') may result.

INFECTIVE ENDOCARDITIS
Acute bacterial endocarditis is usually due to bacteria (e.g. Staphylococci) or fungi affecting previously normal valves in seriously ill patients. Large 'vegetations' cause destruction of the affected valves with murmurs, cardiac failure, septicaemia and widespread infarcts and abscesses due to infected emboli. Treatment is with antibiotics in large doses, but the disease is often fatal.

   Subacute bacterial endocarditis (SABE) is a less severe disease due to *Streptococcus viridans* which attacks previously damaged valves e.g. those affected by rheumatic heart disease.

Clinical features of SABE
1. Heart murmur
2. Fever, weight loss, anaemia
3. Small haemorrhages in the skin (purpura) or nails ('splinter haemorrhages')
4. Finger clubbing
5. Enlarged spleen (splenomegaly)

Treatment
Penicillin in large doses for at least six weeks. To prevent SABE, patients known to have cardiac damage should receive penicillin 'cover' for dental extractions.

SYPHILIS
Tertiary syphilis may cause *aortic incompetence* or *aortic aneurysm*.

Cardiac failure

Heart failure is the inability of the heart to maintain the normal circulation. Either the L. side or the R. side of the heart may fail first, but eventually both sides will be involved.

L. VENTRICULAR FAILURE

Causes
1. Myocardial ischaemia
2. Hypertension
3. Aortic stenosis or incompetence

Clinical features
1. Pulmonary congestion or pulmonary oedema (p. 19)
2. Tachycardia
3. Cardiac enlargement
4. Cyanosis

Treatment of left ventricular failure
Mild cases may be controlled by increased rest, reduction of obesity, avoidance of physical and mental stress, and a regular diuretic (p. 145) with potassium.

Moderate cases may need digitalis and a low-salt diet in addition.

Severe cases may need bed rest with the legs dependent (cardiac bed), high concentration oxygen therapy, and i.v. aminophylline, frusemide and morphine.

The nurse should watch for evidence of digitalis toxicity (p. 145).

R. VENTRICULAR FAILURE

Causes
1. Following L. ventricular failure
2. Mitral stenosis
3. Pulmonary disease e.g. chronic bronchitis
4. Congenital heart disease

Clinical features
1. Tiredness and weakness
2. Digestive disturbances (due to gastrointestinal congestion)
3. Oedema of dependent parts (ankles, sacrum)
4. Increased jugular venous pressure
5. Large tender liver, often with ascites

Treatment of right ventricular failure
This resembles that of left ventricular failure, but morphine should be avoided in patients with pulmonary disease as it causes respiratory depression.

PULMONARY OEDEMA

Causes
1. Left atrial or ventricular failure

2. Severe pneumonia
3. Excess of intravenous fluid
4. Inhalation of irritant gas e.g. chlorine

Clinical features
The patient is orthopnoeic and distressed, usually cyanosed, and coughing up large quantities of white or pink frothy sputum. The pulse is rapid and in severe cases the BP falls and 'shock' ensues.

Treatment
1. High concentration oxygen therapy with patient sitting up with legs dependent
2. Intravenous morphine, frusemide and aminophylline
3. Digitalis

Myocardial ischaemia

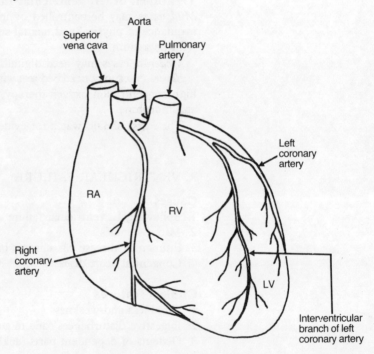

Figure 2.17
Coronary arteries on the surface of the heart

The R. and L. coronary arteries arise from the root of the aorta as soon as it leaves the heart. The right coronary artery supplies the right atrium and the right ventricles, and the left supplies the left atrium and both ventricles. Narrowing of the lumen of these arteries by atheroma or thrombosis leads to myocardial ischaemia which may produce angina or infarction.

Factors predisposing to coronary artery disease
1. Increased blood lipids (? due to high intake of animal fat)
2. Hypertension

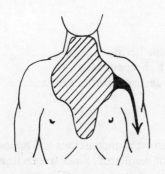

Figure 2.18
Angina. Pain radiates from the
central chest area down the left arm

3. Cigarette smoking
4. Lack of exercise and obesity
5. Diabetes mellitus
6. Family history of myocardial infarction

ANGINA PECTORIS

Crushing substernal pain, usually provoked by effort or emotion and
relieved by rest. It may radiate into the neck or down the L. arm or both
arms. ECG usually shows changes of myocardial ischaemia. Treatment is
with trinitrin (chewed slowly) or a beta-blocker (p. 146) and moderation
of the patient's way of life.

MYOCARDIAL INFARCTION

A plaque of atheroma or a clot in a branch of a coronary artery (*coronary
thrombosis*) may occlude the vessel completely and cause necrosis
(*infarction*) of an area of the myocardium.

Clinical features
1. Sudden angina, which may occur at rest, and persists for hours
2. May be dyspnoea, intense anxiety, syncope or vomiting
3. Pallor or cyanosis, sweating, tachycardia, hypotension

Common complications
1. L. ventricular failure
2. Cardiac arrhythmia or heart block
3. Cardiac arrest
4. 'Shock'
5. Pericarditis
6. Pulmonary embolism (from leg vein thrombosis)
7. Systemic embolism from clot on the infarcted area
8. Rupture or aneurysm of the cardiac wall

Treatment
1. Admission to intensive care unit with constant ECG monitoring and
   facilities to deal with cardiac arrest
2. The patient should rest comfortably in bed and be spared undue
   movement and anxiety
3. Analgesics (e.g. diamorphine or pethidine) should be given as
   necessary
4. Cardiac failure is treated with high conc. oxygen and diuretics
5. Anticoagulants are sometimes used to prevent embolism
6. Drugs such as atropine, lignocaine or phenytoin may be needed to
   treat or prevent arrhythmias
7. If the obstruction to the coronary artery is localized, it may be possible
   to bypass it by using a vein graft taken from the leg.

COMMON CAUSES OF CHEST PAIN
1. Myocardial ischaemia e.g. coronary atheroma, severe anaemia
2. Pericarditis

3. Pleurisy
4. Pulmonary embolism
5. Oesophageal pain e.g. carcinoma, hiatus hernia
6. Pain from chest wall e.g. fractured rib, herpes zoster
7. Pain referred from the abdomen e.g. gastric ulcer or gallstones

Cardiac arrest

This is recognized by the fact that the patient is unconscious and has no carotid pulse. The pupils may or may not be dilated. Since irreversible brain damage occurs within 2–3 minutes the nurse must call for help and start immediate resuscitation, as follows:

1. Make sure the patient is on a firm surface (e.g. floor or fracture boards)
2. Clear the airway (remove dentures and extend the neck)
3. Commence artificial respiration (mouth-to-mouth or Ambu bag, 15 breaths per minute) and external cardiac massage (60 compressions of the sternum per minute)

Remember to close the nostrils and support the jaw during artificial respiration. If resuscitation is effective the pulse should be palpable and the dilated pupils should contract. When help arrives the patient will be intubated and ventilated with oxygen. An i.v. infusion of drugs such as sodium bicarbonate, lignocaine and calcium chloride will be administered and defibrillating shocks will be applied.

Cardiac arrest is due either to cessation of ventricular activity (*cardiac asystole*) or to *ventricular fibrillation*. An ECG is needed to distinguish these two possibilities (see Fig. 2.19) but resuscitation must not be delayed to obtain records.

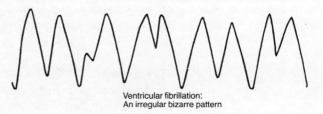

Ventricular fibrillation:
An irregular bizarre pattern

Figure 2.19

Cardiac asystole:
A flat trace

Pericarditis

Inflammation of the pericardium may be *dry* or associated with a fluid *effusion*.

Causes
1. Myocardial infarction
2. 'Benign' pericarditis (usually viral)

3. Bacterial e.g. TB, pneumonia, septicaemia
4. Rheumatic fever
5. Severe uraemia

Clinical features of dry pericarditis
1. Substernal pain, often related to respiration
2. Cough, dyspnoea, pyrexia and tachycardia
3. Pericardial friction rub

Clinical features of pericardial effusion
1. Substernal discomfort and dyspnoea
2. Raised venous pressure
3. Large effusions may reduce the cardiac output
In *chronic constrictive pericarditis* the heart is enclosed by fibrous tissue (often calcified) due to previous TB. This impedes the normal filling of the heart and may need to be removed surgically.

Thrombosis

A blood clot in the heart, arteries or veins.
   The effects of thrombosis vary according to the site, but it may cause blockage of a vessel either at its site of production, or by breaking away to form an embolus which is carried to another area (p. 24). Even a thrombus which is causing no symptoms is potentially dangerous, for there may be further spread of the thrombosis, or an embolus may lodge in a major vessel.

Predisposing factors
1. Damage to lining of the heart or blood-vessel e.g. atheroma
2. Slowing of blood-flow e.g. prolonged bed-rest
3. Increased blood coagulability e.g. oestrogen therapy
Common sites include:
1. Heart
     (i) Left atrium, in mitral stenosis
     (ii) Left ventricle, in myocardial infarction
2. Arteries
     (i) Coronary
     (ii) Cerebral
3. Veins
     (i) Superficial varicose veins in the leg
     (ii) Deep veins of the calf
     (iii) Femoral or iliac veins e.g. in pregnancy
     (iv) Haemorrhoids ('piles')

'Deep-vein thrombosis' (DVT) of the calf
Clinical features
1. Slight pyrexia
2. Pain and tenderness in the calf, worse on dorsiflexion of the foot

3. Oedema of the ankle
4. May be no symptoms until pulmonary embolism occurs

Prevention of DVT
1. Leg exercises, calf massage and early mobilisation
2. Avoidance of anything which impedes venous return from the legs
3. Anticoagulants

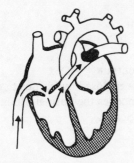

Figure 2.20
Clot from DVT blocking L. pulmonary artery

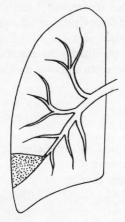

Figure 2.21
Small pulmonary infarction due to a small embolus

Embolism

An *embolus* is a foreign body which is transported from one part of the circulatory system to another, where it becomes impacted. This process is called *embolism*. It cuts off the blood supply to the affected part, which usually produces an area of necrosis called an *infarct*.

Causes of embolism
1. Blood clot (thrombus) from heart or leg veins
2. Air entering veins during operation or due to injury
3. Fat from a fractured bone
4. Clumps of bacteria from heart valves in bacterial endocarditis

Pulmonary embolism occurs when an embolus from the venous circulation reaches the pulmonary arteries or one of their branches in the lungs.

Clinical features depend on the size of the infarct. There may be chest pain, haemoptysis, dyspnoea or sudden death.

Cerebral embolism is usually due to an embolus from the *left* side of the heart. It produces sudden loss of function of a part of the brain, resulting, for example, in coma, paralysis or loss of speech.

Embolism of a limb artery causes a pale or blue limb which may be painful or numb. The pulse in the limb disappears and the limb feels cold to the touch. Unless the circulation is quickly re-established gangrene may result.

Phlebitis (inflammation of a vein). Often occurs in varicose veins, or at a site of injury or infection.

Superficial phlebitis causes pain and redness, and the vein can be felt as a tender cord. The inflammation may cause a clot to form (*thrombophlebitis*).

Special tests in cardiology

1. X-rays
These show the size, shape and position of the heart and great vessels. Even minor degrees of left ventricular failure can be detected radiologically by changes in the lungs.

2. Electrocardiogram
This records the electrical changes taking place in the myocardium during the cardiac cycle. It is particularly valuable in the diagnosis of cardiac arrhythmias and myocardial ischaemia or infarction.

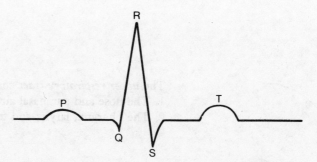

Figure 2.22
The normal electrocardiogram

The P wave is caused by electrical activity in the atria, and the QRS complex results from electrical activity in the ventricles. In atrial fibrillation the P waves disappear.

3. Echo-cardiography
In this technique, ultra-sound is reflected from the heart and recorded electronically, and this gives information about size and shape of the heart chambers and valves.

4. Cardiac catheterization
A long hollow catheter is inserted into a vein and pushed onwards until its tip enters, in successive order, the right atrium, the right ventricle, the pulmonary artery and a small pulmonary arteriole in the lung. At each site the pressure is measured and blood samples are taken for analysis of oxygen and carbon dioxide content. The data about blood flow within the heart which is thus produced allows the site of the anatomical abnormality to be inferred.

5. Ciné-angiography
A suitable radio-opaque dye is injected via the cardiac catheter and X-ray ciné-films are taken which outline the heart chambers and valves.

6. Coronary angiography
In this technique, the opaque dye is injected into the origin of the coronary arteries at the root of the aorta, and blockage or narrowing of the coronary arteries can then be detected on the X-ray screen.

FURTHER READING

Goodland N L 1978 Coronary care, 3rd edn. Wright, Bristol
Hamer J 1978 Introduction to electro-cardiography, 2nd edn. Pitman Medical, London
Julian D G 1978 Cardiology, 3rd edn. Bailliere Tindall, London
Turner P P 1979 Cardiovascular system. Churchill Livingstone, Edinburgh

3 Respiratory system

The *upper respiratory tract* consists of:
1. The nose and paranasal air sinuses
2. The pharynx, larynx and trachea

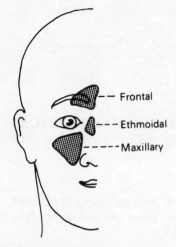

The paranasal air sinuses
The *frontal, ethmoidal* and *maxillary sinuses* are as shown. *The sphenoidal* sinuses lie behind the upper part of the nasal cavity.

Figure 3.1

The *lower respiratory tract* consists of:
1. The bronchi, bronchioles and alveolar ducts
2. The alveoli (air cells) in the lung

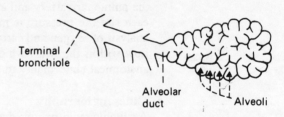

Figure 3.2
The aveoli are surrounded by the pulmonary capillaries.

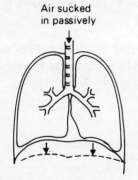

Figure 3.3
The diaphragm is attached to the bottom of the thoracic cage and it flattens as it contracts

Respiration

Respiration allows oxygen (O_2) to be taken up by the tissues and carbon dioxide (CO_2) to be eliminated from the body

External respiration refers to the absorption of O_2 from the air, and the elimination of CO_2 by the lungs. This exchange of gases occurs by diffusion across the alveolar membrane and the capillary endothelium. CO_2 elimination regulates the pH of the blood.

Internal respiration refers to the gaseous exchange between the cells in the various body tissues and their surrounding tissue fluids.

Ventilation (movement of air in and out of the lungs)
This is brought about by changes in size of the thoracic cavity, the lungs following these variations passively. The muscles concerned with

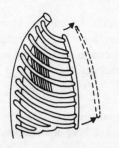

Figure 3.4
The external intercostals elevate the ribs and this pushes the sternum forward

inspiration are the *diaphragm* and the *external intercostals*. The process of breathing is controlled by the *respiratory centre,* a collection of neurones in the medulla of the brain. The respiratory centre is stimulated by an increase in the carbon dioxide content of the blood.

RESPIRATORY RATE

The normal rate is about 12–20 per min in the adult and 40 per min in the infant.

The normal respiration : pulse ratio is about 1 : 4.

Causes of rapid respiration

1. Exertion, excitement or fever
2. Anoxaemia (decreased oxygen content of blood)
3. Pain associated with breathing e.g. pleurisy or peritonitis may cause rapid shallow respiration

Causes of slow respiration

Depression of respiratory centre e.g. terminal illness, head injury, barbiturate overdose

Dyspnoea (a feeling of breathlessness)

Causes
1. Pulmonary or cardiac disease
2. Obstruction to air entry into lungs
3. Acidosis (e.g. renal failure)
4. Psychological (e.g. anxiety)

LUNG VOLUMES

A spirometer can be used to record the volume of air inhaled and exhaled during respiration.

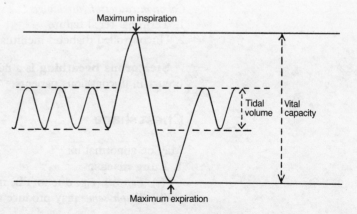

Figure 3.5
Lung volumes

Resting tidal volume: the volume of air breathed in and out in a single quiet respiration at rest (about 500 ml in an adult).

Vital Capacity: the largest volume a subject can expire after a single maximum inspiration (about 4.5 litres in a young adult male). The vital capacity can be reduced in practically any lung disease.

FEV_1 (Forced expiratory volume in one second): the volume expired in one second when, after a maximum inspiration, the expiration is performed as rapidly as possible. This is reduced in obstructive airway disease such as asthma, emphysema and bronchitis.

RESPIRATORY RHYTHM

Inspiration and expiration should take an equal time

Prolonged *inspiration* occurs in laryngeal or tracheal obstruction (e.g. croup)

Prolonged *expiration* occurs in bronchial obstruction (e.g. asthma)

Cheyne-Stokes breathing. The depth of respiration increases progressively to a maximum, then diminishes to a period of apnoea (absent breathing) and the cycle is repeated:

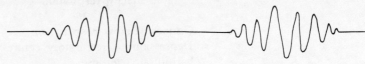

Figure 3.6

This is due to decreased sensitivity of the respiratory centre to CO_2.

Common causes of Cheyne-Stokes breathing
1. Severe cardiac failure
2. Pneumonia
3. Barbiturate overdose
4. Cerebro-vascular accident
5. Head injury

'**Air hunger**' (Kussmaul's breathing) consists of very deep respirations due to stimulation of the respiratory centre by acidosis.

Common causes of 'air hunger'
1. Terminal renal failure
2. Uncontrolled diabetes mellitus

Stertorous breathing is a noisy snoring type of respiration which occurs in unconscious patients.

Chest shape

May be abnormal in:
1. **Lung disease**
   (i) *Fibrosis* (e.g. due to TB) may flatten the affected area
   (ii) *Emphysema* may produce a barrel-shaped chest

2. **Bone disease**
   (i) *Spinal kyphosis* (anterior bending) or *scoliosis* (lateral bending) may restrict lung movement
   (ii) *Rickets* may cause flattening of the rib cage due to bending of the soft ribs

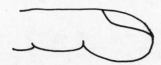

Figure 3.7

Clubbing

A bulbous enlargement of the terminal phalanges, with curved nails and filling-in of the angle at the nail base

Causes
1. Bronchial carcinoma
2. Chronic pulmonary suppuration
3. Bacterial endocarditis
4. Cyanotic congenital heart disease

Cough and sputum

Types of cough, and their causes
1. *Dry* (without sputum)
    (i) Diseases of throat, larynx or trachea
    (ii) Early stages of pneumonia
    (iii) Psychological ('nervous' cough)
2. *Productive* (with sputum)
    (i) Bronchitis
    (ii) TB
    (iii) Pneumonia
    (iv) Bronchiectasis or lung abscess
3. *Spasmodic* (a series of explosive coughs)
    (i) Whooping cough
    (ii) 'Croup'
4. *'Brassy'* (characteristic noise due to pressure on the trachea)
   Aortic aneurysm

Types of sputum
1. *Mucoid* (clear or white)
    (i) Chronic bronchitis
    (ii) Asthma
   In asthma there may be sticky plugs ('casts' of the bronchial tree)
2. *Purulent* (yellow or green)
   May occur with any lung infection. In bronchiectasis and lung abscess the sputum is often copious and foul-smelling
3. *Haemoptysis* (blood-stained)
    (i) Pulmonary disease e.g. bronchial carcinoma, TB
    (ii) Cardiac disease e.g. mitral stenosis
   In lobar pneumonia the sputum may be rust-coloured
4. *Pink, frothy and copious*
   Pulmonary oedema

Microscopic examination of the sputum may reveal *bacteria* (e.g. in bronchitis, TB or pneumonia), *eosinophils* (in allergic asthma) or *malignant cells* (in bronchial carcinoma).

   Culture of the sputum enables bacteria to be identified, and their sensitivity to various antibiotics to be tested.

Bronchitis

Inflammation of the bronchial mucosa

ACUTE BRONCHITIS

Causes
1. Downward spread of upper respiratory infection e.g. coryza or sinusitis
2. Systemic viral infection e.g. measles or influenza
3. Irritant gases e.g. 'smog' or smoke

Clinical features
1. Pyrexia
2. Central chest soreness
3. Cough, with or without sputum
4. Dyspnoea and wheezing with cyanosis in severe cases

Complications
1. Secondary bacterial infection is very common
2. Bronchopneumonia
3. Cardiac failure, especially in the elderly

Treatment
1. Bed rest in a warm room with steam inhalations
2. Antibiotics such as tetracycline or penicillin
3. Codeine linctus to suppress troublesome cough

CHRONIC BRONCHITIS

Predisposing causes
1. Air pollution (i.e. urban environment)
2. Cigarette smoking
3. Dirty or dusty occupations
4. Obesity

Clinical features
1. 'Smokers' cough with early morning sputum
2. Later a 'winter' cough develops, with wheezing and sputum which may be mucoid or purulent. These symptoms gradually become more persistent
3. Progressively increasing dyspnoea, with cyanosis

Complications
1. Cor pulmonale (i.e. heart failure secondary to lung disease) with recurrent episodes of right ventricular failure
2. Bronchopneumonia

Treatment
1. Avoidance of cigarette smoking, dusty work and obesity

2. Bronchodilators e.g. salbutamol
3. Antibiotics such as tetracycline or ampicillin should be given if the sputum becomes purulent
4. Sedative cough mixtures e.g. codeine linctus, will suppress cough at night. Expectorant cough mixtures may loosen sputum
5. Low concentration oxygen therapy for severe cases

Emphysema

A lung disease in which there is enlargement of the alveoli with destruction of their walls. Usually occurs in association with chronic bronchitis or chronic asthma. Patients are dyspnoeic on exertion, with a barrel-shaped chest which expands poorly.

Pneumonias

In pneumonia, alveolar inflammation causes the affected lung to become airless and solid with exudate (*consolidation*).

Organisms which commonly cause pneumonia
1. Streptococcus pneumoniae (pneumococcus)
2. Haemophilus influenzae
3. Mycobacterium tuberculosis (TB)
4. Staphylococcus aureus
5. Mycoplasma and viruses

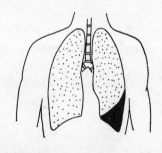

Figure 3.8
Consolidation (lobar pneumonia). The affected area is dull to percussion, and the alveoli are airlesss

LOBAR PNEUMONIA
This is localized to one or more lobes of the lungs. Pneumococcus is the commonest causative organism, and it often affects previously healthy adults.

Clinical features of lobar pneumonia
1. Sudden onset of pyrexia and rigors or vomiting
2. Dyspnoea, with rapid shallow respiration and cyanosis
3. Cough with 'rusty' sputum
4. Pleuritic pain (worse on cough and deep breathing)
5. Herpes labialis (vesicles on lips due to herpes simplex virus)

Complications
1. Pleural effusion
2. Empyema
3. Cardiac failure
4. Septicaemia

BRONCHOPNEUMONIA
This has a more patchy distribution and spreads along the bronchioles. It is due to a variety of organisms (especially Haemophilus) and is often secondary to other disease. Young children and the elderly are most commonly affected.

Predisposing causes
1. Bronchitis
2. Inhalation of infected material (e.g. mucus) or vomitus
3. Debilitation, with recumbency and poor respiratory movements
4. Pulmonary embolism or collapse

Clinical features
Resembles lobar pneumonia, but the onset is more gradual, cough and sputum are more variable, and pyrexia is irregular and resolves gradually.

Complications
1. Cardiac failure
2. Pulmonary fibrosis

Treatment of bacterial pneumonia
1. Antibiotics according to bacterial sensitivity e.g. i.m. benzyl-penicillin for pneumococcus
2. Pleuritic pain may require pethidine
3. Codeine will suppress irritant cough
4. High concentration oxygen therapy if central cyanosis develops

Bronchiectasis

This is a localized dilation of the bronchi, usually accompanied by recurrent bronchial suppuration in the affected lobes.

Causes
1. Complication of pulmonary collapse
2. Complication of pneumonia, especially TB or bronchopneumonia

Clinical features
1. Cough with profuse purulent sputum, especially on changing posture
2. Malaise, intermittent pyrexia, halitosis ('bad breath')
3. Weight loss (or 'failure to thrive' in a child)
4. Dyspnoea, often with cyanosis
5. Finger clubbing
6. Some patients have no symptoms

Complications
1. Recurrent pneumonia or pleurisy
2. Lung abscess or empyema
3. Septic emboli

Treatment
1. Frequent postural drainage
2. Antibiotics
3. Surgical removal of the affected lobe

Industrial lung diseases

Pneumoconiosis is chronic lung disease due to inhalation of dusts by industrial workers.

Types of pneumoconiosis

1. *Anthracosis*, in coal mines
2. *Silicosis*, in sand-blasters
3. *Siderosis*, in iron miners and foundry workers
4. *Asbestosis*, in workers with asbestos

Clinical features

Progressive dyspnoea, with cough and sputum

Complications

1. Pulmonary fibrosis
2. Emphysema
3. Cor pulmonale (cardiac failure secondary to lung disease)
4. Some types predispose to TB or cancer

Treatment

1. Avoidance of the dust
2. As for chronic bronchitis (p. 30)

Asthma

Intermittent bronchial spasm, often accompanied by sticky bronchial secretions. A severe attack lasting for many hours is called *status asthmaticus*.

Predisposing causes

1. Many patients have an *atopic constitution* with a family history of asthma, infantile eczema, urticaria or hay fever. Such patients are often allergic to mites, pollens, animal hair, certain foods etc.
2. *Chronic bronchitis* and *respiratory tract infections*
3. *Psychological factors* e.g. stress at work, or tension in the home
4. Many cases develop in middle-age for no apparent cause (*idiopathic*)

Clinical features

1. Paroxysms of dyspnoea, with 'tightness' in the chest, and prolonged wheezy expirations
2. Cough (dry or with sticky plugs of sputum)
3. In severe cases, cyanosis and respiratory failure

Complications

1. Emphysema may develop in long-standing asthmatics
2. Recurrent chest infections

Treatment
1. *Antispasmodics* (drugs which relax the bronchial muscles)
   (i) Aminophylline by i.v. injection or suppository
   (ii) Isoprenaline
       Orciprenaline *(Alupent)*
       Salbutamol *(Ventolin)* } by tablet or aerosol inhalers

   The excessive use of isoprenaline aerosols can cause death and patients must not exceed the recommended dose.
2. *Corticosteroids*
   ACTH, prednisone or hydrocortisone (p. 149) may be needed in severe cases. *Becotide Inhaler* delivers a potent glucocorticoid to the lungs with no danger of systemic side-effects.
3. *Sodium cromoglycate (Intal)*
   This may be administered regularly by a 'Spinhaler' to prevent asthma by inhibiting the release of bronchoconstrictor substances.
4. *Antibiotics* e.g. tetracycline
   These are used only if the sputum is infected.
5. *Oxygen therapy in low concentration* (p. 34)
6. *Avoidance of allergens*
   House dust mites etc. should be removed from the environment by frequent use of a vacuum cleaner. In some cases desensitizing injections may help.

Oxygen therapy

This is used to correct tissue *hypoxia* (low oxygen tension).

High concentration oxygen therapy (40–80 per cent)
This is indicated in central cyanosis due to impaired gas exchange:
1. Shock e.g. myocardial infarction
2. Pulmonary oedema
3. Pneumonia
4. Cardiac failure (other than cor pulmonale, p. 18)
   Suitable masks: Polymask or MC mask (Henley)

Low concentration oxygen therapy (25–40 per cent)
This is indicated in underventilation of the lungs due to chronic respiratory disease:
1. Chronic bronchitis
2. Emphysema
3. Severe, prolonged asthma
   Suitable masks: Ventimask or Edinburgh mask
   The administration of high conc. oxygen to a patient with carbon dioxide retention due to chronic respiratory disease may release the respiratory centre of the brain from its 'anoxic drive' and cause respiratory depression, with coma due to carbon dioxide narcosis. Only low conc. oxygen should be used in chronic respiratory disease.

Tuberculosis

In developed countries infection is with the human TB bacillus (*Mycobacterium tuberculosis*) which spreads by droplet infection in the atmosphere and affects the lungs.

In under-developed countries infection with the bovine TB bacillus also occurs. This is transmitted in milk and causes TB of the intestine.

Primary TB is infection with the tubercle bacillus in a patient who has not previously been infected.

Post-primary TB is re-infection or a recrudescence of the primary lesion.

These 2 conditions follow different courses due to the increased immunological response in the post-primary disease.

PRIMARY TB

A small lesion occurs in any part of the lungs and the local hilar lymph nodes enlarge. The *Mantoux test* (intradermal injection of tuberculin) becomes positive. Most primary lesions heal spontaneously without complications, but occasionally pleural effusion or tuberculous bronchopneumonia may develop.

When tuberculosis spreads to the cervical lymph nodes they may enlarge and break down to form an abscess. This produces a soft, fluctuant swelling which is not usually hot or tender, and so it is called a 'cold abscess'. This may need to be drained surgically.

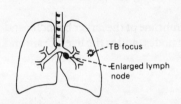

TB focus
Enlarged lymph node

Figure 3.9

POST-PRIMARY PULMONARY TB

The initial lesion is usually in the upper lobe of the lung but spread into other parts of the lung often follows. Necrosis of the affected part (*caseation*) may produce a cavity. The course is variable, depending on the patient's resistance. Healing may occur with fibrosis and calcification, but the disease usually slowly progresses unless halted by treatment.

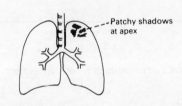

Patchy shadows at apex

Figure 3.10

Clinical features
1. Early cases may have no symptoms
2. Malaise, pyrexia, anorexia, weight loss, tiredness or night sweats
3. Cough, may be dry or productive, sometimes with haemoptysis
4. In advanced cases, dyspnoea, cyanosis and wasting (cachexia)

Complications
1. Widespread tuberculous bronchopneumonia
2. Pleurisy, often with effusion or empyema
3. Massive haemoptysis
4. Blood-borne spread to another organ e.g. bone, meninges or kidney
5. Miliary TB (widespread dissemination throughout the body)

Treatment
1. Long-term chemotherapy with drugs such as rifampicin, isoniazid and ethambutol, given in combination to prevent the emergence of resistant organisms

2. Adequate diet and rest
3. Surgical resection of affected lung in selected cases

Prevention
1. Improved hygiene and living conditions
2. Detection and isolation of patients with 'open' TB (i.e. bacilli in the sputum)
3. Vaccination with an attenuated strain of bacillus (BCG)

Lung tumours

1. BRONCHIAL CARCINOMA
This is the second commonest cancer in Britain. (Skin cancer is the commonest.)

It usually arises from the mucous membrane of the larger bronchi, and it spreads early to the mediastinal lymph nodes, and to the liver, brain and bone.

Predisposing causes
1. Cigarette smoking is by far the most important
2. Atmospheric pollution

Clinical features
1. Cough, which may be dry or productive
2. Weight loss, malaise, anorexia
3. Chest pain, dyspnoea, haemoptysis

Common complications
1. Bronchial obstruction, with pulmonary collapse or infection (pneumonia or abscess)
2. Pleural effusion, often blood-stained
3. Obstruction of superior vena cava
4. Distant metastasis (spread to other organs)

Treatment
1. Surgical resection of the affected lung
2. Radiotherapy or cytotoxic drugs in selected cases

2. SECONDARY CARCINOMA
Cancer of other organs (e.g. breast) commonly spreads to the lungs (*pulmonary metastases*). It usually produces small round opacities on the chest x-ray.

3. BENIGN TUMOURS
These are uncommon (e.g. bronchial adenoma), but they may cause haemoptysis or bronchial obstruction.

Pleurisy

Inflammation of the pleura (the membrane which covers the lungs and lines the thoracic cavity) is called pleurisy.

Pleurisy may be *dry* or associated with an *effusion* of fluid. The fluid may be serous (clear, straw-coloured), purulent or blood-stained. A collection of pus in the pleural cavity is called an *empyema*.

Causes of pleurisy

1. Acute infectious fevers, especially respiratory viruses
2. As a complication of pneumonia (especially lobar pneumonia or TB) or lung abscess
3. Bronchial cancer
4. Pulmonary infarction

Clinical features

Dry pleurisy causes pain aggravated by cough and deep breathing. A pleural friction rub may be heard with the stethoscope. If *effusion* occurs the pain disappears but dyspnoea increases.

Treatment of pleurisy

1. Bed rest, with splinting of the ribs by adhesive plaster if necessary to relieve pain
2. Analgesic and cough suppressant (codeine has both properties)
3. Treatment of the underlying cause

Pleural effusion

Causes of pleural effusion

1. Any cause of pleurisy
2. Accompanying generalised fluid retention in severe cardiac, hepatic or renal failure

Treatment of pleural effusion

Pleural tap (Paracentesis)

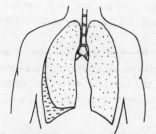

Figure 3.11
Pleural effusion. The affected area is dull to percussion

Pneumothorax

Air in the pleural cavity

Causes

1. Traumatic
2. Iatrogenic e.g. during thoracic surgery
3. Spontaneous
   (i) In previous healthy young adults
   (ii) As a complication of emphysema or asthma

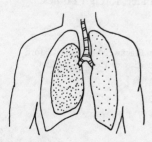

Figure 3.12
Pneumothorax. The affected area is hyper-resonant to percussion. The mediastinum has been displaced to the opposite side

Clinical features

1. Pain in the chest, and dyspnoea
2. With a large pneumothorax the patient may be 'shocked'

3. The affected side is hyper-resonant to percussion, with diminished chest movement. The mediastinum may be pushed to the opposite side.

Treatment
1. Patients who are shocked or in pain may need morphine
2. If the lung is collapsed a catheter is inserted into the pleural cavity, and connected to an under-water seal

Special tests in pulmonary disease

1. Spirometry (p. 27)

2. Arterial blood gases
The overall efficiency of the lungs and the pulmonary circulation can be assessed by measuring the partial pressures of oxygen (p O_2) and carbon dioxide (p CO_2) in the arterial blood.

Normal values at rest: oxygen 80–110 mm mercury
carbon dioxide 36–44 mm mercury

Patients with respiratory obstruction usually have an increased p CO_2, but a decrease in p O_2 is a later, and more serious, finding.

3. Radiology
A *plain chest X-ray* (postero-anterior and lateral) yields much information about the heart, lungs and thoracic cage.

A *tomogram* consists of serial X-ray pictures of a small area, specially focused at different depths to show the detail of a particular shadow seen on a plain X-ray.

A *bronchogram* is used to outline the bronchi (e.g. for suspected bronchiectasis). A small quantity of radio-opaque dye, injected via a nasal catheter into the trachea, is inhaled into the bronchi with the patient positioned so that the dye drains into the suspect area, which is then X-rayed.

4. Bronchoscopy
In this technique an illuminated rigid tube is passed through the larynx and trachea into the bronchi. It may be used to inspect and biopsy bronchial tumours, and also to remove inhaled foreign bodies.

FURTHER READING

Brewis R A L 1975 Lecture notes on respiratory disease. Blackwell Scientific, Oxford
Cole R B 1975 Essentials of respiratory disease, 2nd edn. Pitman Medical, London

4

Digestive system

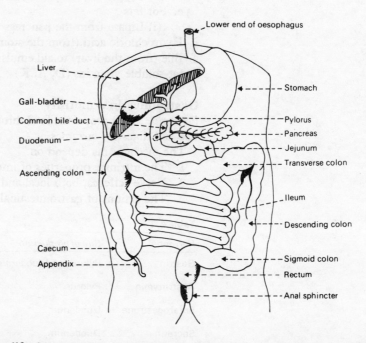

Lower end of oesophagus

Liver

Gall-bladder

Common bile-duct

Duodenum

Ascending colon

Caecum

Appendix

Stomach

Pylorus

Pancreas

Jejunum

Transverse colon

Ileum

Descending colon

Sigmoid colon

Rectum

Anal sphincter

Figure 4.1
Gastrointestinal tract from lower
oesophagus to anus

In life the transverse colon lies just below the liver and in front of the pylorus

Digestion and absorption

The function of the gastrointestinal tract is to digest and absorb the following nutrients:
1. Carbohydrate, protein and fat
2. Vitamins
3. Minerals (especially sodium, calcium and iron)
4. Water

DIGESTION
Digestion (the breaking down of food into absorbable units) begins in the mouth and stomach and is completed in the small intestine.

Requirements for digestion
1. Mastication (chewing) and normal gastro-intestinal motility (q.v.)
2. Digestive enzymes
  a. For carbohydrates
    (i) Amylase (ptyalin) from the salivary glands

(ii) Amylase from the pancreas

(iii) Maltase and lactase from the small intestine

b. For proteins

(i) Pepsin from the stomach

(ii) Trypsin and chymotrypsin from the pancreas

c. For fats

(i) Lipase from the pancreas

3. Hydrochloric acid (from the stomach) to activate pepsin

4. Bile (from the liver) to aid emulsification and absorption of fats and fat-soluble vitamins (D, A, K)

Gastrointestinal motility

Peristaltic waves propel the food through the intestine and mix it with the bile and digestive enzymes.

The mechanisms depend on:

1. The intrinsic properties of intestinal smooth muscle

2. Nerve reflexes, both local and via the brain

3. The actions of gastrointestinal hormones (shown below)

Table 4.1

Hormone	Site of production	Action
Gastrin	Pylorus and duodenum	Stimulates gastric acid secretion
Gastrozymin	Pylorus	Stimulates gastric enzyme secretion
Enterogastrone	Duodenum	Inhibits gastric secretion
Secretin	Duodenum	Stimulates watery secretion by the pancreas
Pancreozymin	Duodenum	Stimulates enzyme secretion by the pancreas
Cholecystokinin	Duodenum	Stimulates gall-bladder contraction

These hormones affect both digestive enzyme secretion and G.I. secretion and G.I. motility. Their actions overlap and interact in a complex way.

ABSORPTION

The products of digestion are as follows:

1. Carbohydrates are broken down to three *monosaccharides* (glucose, galactose and fructose)

2. Proteins are broken down to *amino-acids*

3. Fats are broken down to *fatty acids and glycerol*

The absorptive surface of the small intestine is greatly increased by finger-like processes called *villi*. Each villus contains a network of *capillaries* and a blind-ended lymphatic (*lacteal*).

The capillaries absorb monosaccharides, amino-acids, minerals and water-soluble vitamins, and these are transported by the portal vein to the liver. The lacteals absorb digested fats and fat-soluble vitamins (D, A and K) and these are transported via the thoracic duct to the bloodstream.

Water, sodium and chloride are absorbed in the colon.

VITAMINS

Vitamins are complex chemicals, found in food in very small quantities, which are essential for health and development.

Infants, pregnant women, alcoholics and elderly people living alone are particularly likely to develop a vitamin deficiency.

Multiple vitamin deficiency with protein deprivation is common in developing countries, but it is unusual in the U.K. unless there is another factor such as alcoholism, malabsorption or a food fad.

Vitamin A occurs in animal fats, eggs and carrots. Deficiency causes night blindness and dry painful eyes.

Vitamin B complex occurs in eggs, peas, beans and cereals.

1. *Thiamine* deficiency, which occurs where polished rice is the staple diet, causes *beri-beri* (heart failure and neuropathy)
2. *Riboflavine* deficiency causes sore *lips and tongue*
3. *Nicotinamide* deficiency occurs in the tropics and causes *pellagra* (diarrhoea, dementia and dermatitis)
4. *Cyanocobalamin* (B_{12}) deficiency causes *megaloblastic anaemic* and *subacute combined degeneration of the cord* (p. 111)

Vitamin C (ascorbic acid) occurs in fresh vegetables, especially citrus fruits, but it is destroyed by heat. Deficiency causes scurvy (anaemia, bleeding tendency, spongy gums and delayed healing).

Vitamin D (calciferol)

See page 129.

Vitamin K is found in green vegetables, and is also synthesized by bacteria in the intestine.

Deficiency causes bleeding due to lack of clotting factors (prothrombin and factor 7).

Folic acid occurs in many foods. It is necessary for normal cell division, and folate deficiency results in macrocytic anaemia.

The mouth and pharynx

The tongue

Pallor indicates anaemia

Dry brown tongue may occur in any severe illness, especially uraemia and acute intestinal obstruction

'Furring' may be due to smoking, or to many mild illnesses, especially gastrointestinal upsets

Smooth, red tongue (atrophic glossitis) may be due to antibiotics, anaemia or vitamin deficiency

White patches may be due to Candidiasis (p. 124) or leukoplakia (thickened epithelium)

Causes of stomatitis (inflammation of the mouth)
1. Debilitation, excessive smoking, alcoholism
2. Infections
   (i) Viral e.g. measles, herpes simplex
   (ii) Bacterial e.g. pyorrhoea
   (iii) Candidiasis ('thrush')

3. Iron or vitamin deficiency

Mouth toilet is especially important in denture-wearers and in dehydrated patients.

Causes of dysphagia (difficulty in swallowing)
1. Painful conditions of mouth or pharynx e.g. stomatitis, tonsillitis
2. Paralysis of muscles of pharynx e.g. poliomyelitis
3. Foreign body in the oesophagus or pharynx
4. Disease of the oesophagus e.g. cancer
5. Compression of oesophagus e.g. by thyroid or bronchial cancer

N.B. For examination purposes, whenever you are asked to mention causes of failure of passage along a tube (e.g. food along the oesophagus) it is worth considering the following:

1. Failure of propulsion

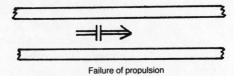

Figure 4.2

Failure of propulsion

2. Blockage in the lumen e.g. foreign body

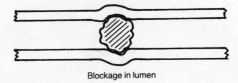

Figure 4.3

Blockage in lumen

3. Blockage from a lesion in the wall

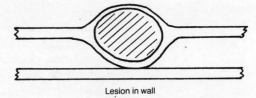

Figure 4.4

Lesion in wall

4. Blockage from a lesion outside the wall

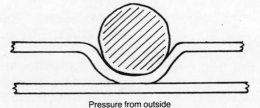

Figure 4.5

Pressure from outside

The stomach

Functions of the stomach
1. Storage of food after a meal
2. Mixing of food with gastric secretions
3. Controlled release of the resulting mixture (chyme) into the duodenum
4. Secretion of pepsin
5. Secretion of hydrochloric acid
6. Secretion of intrinsic factor, an enzyme necessary for B_{12} absorption in the terminal ileum

Common causes of anorexia (loss of appetite)
1. Malignancy
2. Gastrointestinal disorders e.g. gastritis
3. Cardiac, hepatic or renal failure
4. Drugs, e.g. digoxin
5. Depression or anxiety
6. Chronic illness, especially if painful

Causes of vomiting
1. *Feeding upsets*: (in babies) and *dietary indiscretions*
2. *Intra-abdominal disease*
   (i) Inflammation
       e.g. Gastric ulcer
            Gastroenteritis
            Peritonitis
            Pancreatitis
            Cholecystitis
            Hepatitis
   (ii) Obstruction (p. 49)
3. *Cerebral*
   (i) Motion sickness
   (ii) Migraine
   (iii) Labyrinthitis
   (iv) Raised intra-cranial pressure
4. *Psychological* e.g. disgust, fear, pain
5. *Metabolic*
   (i) Pregnancy
   (ii) Febrile illness e.g. tonsillitis (especially in children)
   (iii) Uncontrolled diabetes

Types of vomitus
1. Food, usually partly digested
2. Fluid, which may be bile-stained (greeny-black)
3. Blood (haematemesis)
   — bright red if recent
     dark brown ('coffee-grounds') if old

4. Faeculent — dark brown, foul-smelling fluid due to prolonged intestinal obstruction

Projectile vomiting, in which the gastric contents are ejected with great force, occurs in pyloric stenosis.

Causes of haematemesis
1. Peptic ulcer or gastritis
2. Aspirin ingestion
3. Oesophageal varices (dilated veins due to portal hypertension)
4. Hiatus hernia

HIATUS HERNIA
A portion of the upper end of the stomach protrudes through the oesophageal opening of the diaphragm into the thorax.

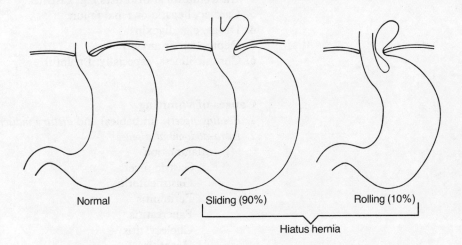

Normal   Sliding (90%)   Rolling (10%)

Hiatus hernia

Figure 4.6

Causes
1. Obesity (due to increased intra-abdominal pressure)
2. Weakness of diaphragmatic muscle in old age

Clinical features
1. Dyspepsia (q.v.), especially on lying down. The reflux of gastric juice attacks the oesophagus and causes oesophagitis
2. Bleeding may cause haematemesis or anaemia

Treatment
1. Weight reduction
2. Small meals and antacids
3. Sleeping in 'head-up' position
4. In severe cases, surgical repair of the diaphragm

DYSPEPSIA
Dyspepsia or 'indigestion' refers to pain, discomfort or passage of wind which is related to the taking of food.

Causes
1. Defective teeth, hurried or irregular meals
2. Dietary indiscretion (excess alcohol, pickles, etc.)
3. Organic disease
   (i) Hiatus hernia
   (ii) Gastritis or gastric carcinoma
   (iii) Peptic ulcer
   (iv) Disease of liver or gall-bladder
   (v) Heart failure

Clinical features
1. Flatulence (epigastric discomfort, distension and belching)
2. Heart-burn (pain behind the sternum)
3. Water-brash (regurgitation of fluid into the mouth)
4. Nausea and vomiting

Treatment
1. Antacids such as aluminium hydroxide or magnesium trisilicate give symptomatic relief
2. Treatment of the underlying cause

Peptic ulcer

GASTRIC ULCER (G.U.)

Clinical features
1. Epigastric pain, usually localized, and occurring soon after food
2. Vomiting, which often relieves the pain
3. Epigastric tenderness

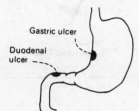

Gastric ulcer

Duodenal ulcer

Figure 4.7
The common sites for peptic ulcer

DUODENAL ULCER (D.U.)

Clinical features resemble gastric ulcer but:
1. The pain may wake the patient in the night and is relieved by food
2. Vomiting is less common in duodenal ulcer
3. Duodenal ulcer is more common in men

Complications of peptic ulcers

1. Bleeding
   Massive haematemesis may cause collapse
   Small bleeds may cause anaemia
2. Perforation
3. Obstruction due to scarring ('hour glass stomach')
4. Gastrocolic fistula (in G.U.)
5. Pyloric stenosis (in D.U.)

The gastric contents accumulate and cause distension of the stomach, which may 'splash' when the stomach is palpated. There is often *projectile vomiting*, in which food eaten hours or even days previously is very forcibly ejected

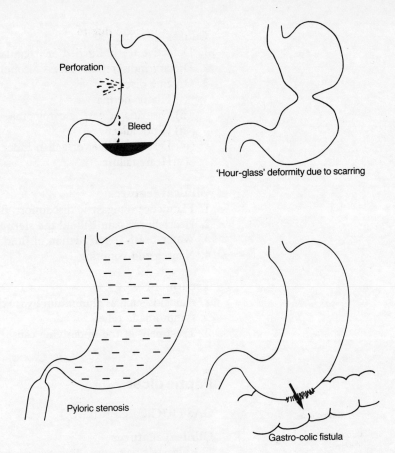

Figure 4.8
Complications of peptic ulcer

Medical treatment of peptic ulcers
1. Adequate rest and removal of anxiety
2. Stop smoking and avoid aspirins
3. Antacids e.g. magnesium trisilicate or aluminium hydroxide
4. Anticholinergic drugs (to diminish gastric peristalsis) e.g. propantheline
5. Carbenoxelone ('Biogastrone' for gastric ulcer; 'Duogastrone' for duodenal ulcer) speeds healing
6. Dietary modification where necessary

FAECES
These normally consist of unabsorbed food residue, bacteria and water

1. Quantity
Copious stools occur in malabsorption
Scanty stools occur in dehydration

2. Colour
The normal brown colour is due to bile pigments.

Pale stools are due to
  (i) Biliary tract obstruction
 (ii) Excessive fat (malabsorption)
Dark grey stools occur after iron ingestion
Black tarry stools (melaena) are due to bleeding in the upper gastrointestinal tract
Red blood in the stools is seen in bleeding from the colon or rectum (e.g. ulcerative colitis, cancer of colon or haemorrhoids)
Pus in the stools occurs in colitis, dysentery and burst pelvic abscess

3. Consistency
Liquid stools occur in diarrhoea
Hard lumpy stools occur in constipation
Slimy stools (due to mucus) occur in diseases of the colon
Foreign bodies or *parasites* such as roundworms, threadworms and tapeworms may also be noted

4. Odour
Very malodorous stools occur in malabsorption

Some characteristic abnormal stools:
1. Malabsorption
Soft, pale, bulky stools, often oily, malodorous and difficult to flush away
2. Dysentery
Watery stools mixed with red blood and pus
3. Cholera
Pale watery stools, free of odour, with shreds of epithelium and mucus ('Rice-water')
4. Intussusception
'Red-currant jelly'

DIARRHOEA
Frequent passage of unformed motions

Causes

Acute
1. Dietary indiscretion e.g. excessive beer
2. Food poisoning e.g. toadstools, Staphylococcal toxins
3. Gastrointestinal infection
   (i) Viral 'gastro-enteritis'
  (ii) Bacterial e.g. typhoid fever or bacillary dysentery
 (iii) Protozoal e.g. amoebic dysentery
4. Psychogenic e.g. nervousness
5. Drugs e.g. purgatives and antibiotics

Chronic
1. Intestinal inflammation
    (i) Ulcerative colitis
    (ii) Diverticulitis
    (iii) Carcinoma of colon
2. Malabsorption (q.v.)
3. Metabolic e.g. thyrotoxicosis

'*Spurious*' diarrhoea can follow the impaction of solid faeces in the elderly. These hard masses may sometimes not respond even to an enema, and they may need to be removed by a gloved finger.

MALABSORPTION

Malabsorption is the defective absorption of one or more dietary components from the gut. Patients with malabsorption may thus suffer from deficiency of protein, fat, carbohydrate, vitamins (especially folic acid) or mineral salts (especially calcium or iron). The patient usually has diarrhoea, and the unabsorbed fat in the faeces makes the stools pale, bulky and malodorous, and since they float they are difficult to flush away. Malabsorption of fat is called *steatorrhoea*, and it can be confirmed by a 3 day stool collection for faecal fat estimation.

The various deficiencies in malabsorption may cause weight loss (or stunted growth in children), anaemia, osteomalacia, tetany or a rash.

Causes
1. Gastrectomy or removal of part of the ileum
2. Biliary tract obstruction
3. Pancreatic failure (chronic pancreatitis or fibrocystic disease)
4. Coeliac disease (flat jejunal mucosa due to gluten allergy)
    In this condition the intestinal villi eventually become flattened so that they lose their absorptive capacity

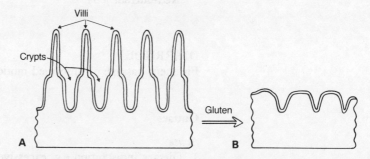

Figure 4.9

(A) Normal jejunum. Digested food is absorbed via crypts and villi

(B) Jejunum in coeliac disease. Mucosal surface is flattened

5. 'Blind-loop' syndrome
    Some intestinal operations, such as the Polya partial gastrectomy leave a 'blind' loop of bowel which becomes filled with bacteria. These may utilize the nutrients in the diet for their own metabolism.

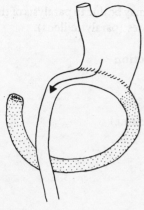

Figure 4.10
'Blind-loop' syndrome. Bacteria
multiply in the stippled area

Treatment of malabsorption
1. Sometimes the deficiency can be corrected by giving oral supplements of iron, calcium, folic acid etc.
2. The underlying cause must be identified and treated if possible: e.g.
    (i) coeliac patients require a strict gluten-free diet (i.e. rigorous exclusion of all wheat products)
    (ii) pancreatic enzyme deficiency is overcome by sprinkling an oral pancreatic preparation on every meal
    (iii) the 'blind-loop' syndrome is treated by an antibiotic such as metronidazole

ABDOMINAL COLIC
'Griping' abdominal pain due to spasmodic contraction of the intestine.

Causes
1. Indigestible foods e.g. unripe apples
2. Gastroenteritis
3. 'Irritable bowel' syndrome ('functional')
4. Intestinal obstruction
5. Purgatives and poisons

CONSTIPATION
Delay in evacuation of faeces.

Many patients are unduly worried about constipation. Many normal people defaecate only once in three days, others as often as three times daily.

Causes
Acute
1. Paralytic ileus
    (i) Abdominal surgery
    (ii) Peritonitis
    (iii) Acute febrile illness (e.g. pneumonia)
2. Obstruction (q.v.)

Chronic
1. Ineffective peristalsis
    (i) Dehydration or lack of solid food
    (ii) Chronic purgation
    (iii) Metabolic e.g. hypothyroidism
    (iv) Drugs e.g. codeine
2. Obstruction (q.v.)
3. Dyschezia (distended insensitive rectum due to persistent failure to respond to the desire to defaecate)

INTESTINAL OBSTRUCTION
This is an obstruction to the peristaltic passage of the intestinal contents along the gut.

The obstruction may be mechanical, or it may be due to paralysis of the intestinal movements so that peristalsis ceases (paralytic ileus).

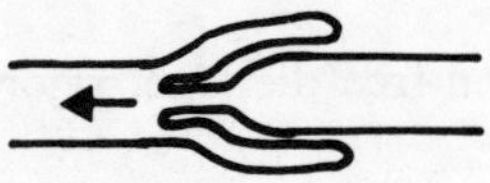

Figure 4.11
Intussusception

Common causes of mechanical obstruction
1. Adhesions from previous operation
2. Strangulated hernia
3. Volvulus (twisted intestine)
4. Intussusception (invagination of the intestine)
5. Tumour e.g. carcinoma of colon

Common causes of paralytic ileus
1. After abdominal surgery
2. Peritonitis

Clinical features of intestinal obstruction
1. Absolute constipation of faeces and flatus
2. Vomiting and consequent dehydration (as shown by dry mouth and inelastic skin)
3. Distended abdomen

In *mechanical* obstruction there is also:
   (i) Severe colicky pain
   (ii) Loud bowel sounds on auscultation of the abdomen

In *paralytic ileus*, by contrast,
   (i) Discomfort is more generalised
   (ii) Bowel sounds are absent

Treatment of intestinal obstruction
1. Naso-gastric suction to prevent vomiting and control distension
2. Intravenous fluids until rehydrated
3. If the cause is mechanical, surgery may be needed

ASCITES
Fluid accumulation in the peritoneal cavity

In this condition the abdomen is distended and the flanks are full to percussion. When the patient rolls over the fluid moves, and this is called 'shifting dullness'.

Causes
1. Peritoneal inflammation
   (i) Secondary cancer deposits
   (ii) TB
2. Increased pressure in portal vein
   (i) Cirrhosis
   (ii) Congestive heart failure
   (iii) Constrictive pericarditis
3. Generalized oedema e.g. nephrotic syndrome

Treatment of ascites
Paracentesis abdominis: under local anaesthetic, a trocar is inserted into

the dull flank and the fluid is *slowly* allowed to drain off. Rapid drainage can cause collapse of the patient.

ACUTE GASTROENTERITIS
The severity of this condition may vary according to the cause from a mild 'tummy upset' in an individual patient to a severe epidemic which may affect many people and can be fatal.

Causes
1. Ingestion of bacterial toxins e.g. Staphylococcal
2. Ingestion of poisons e.g. toadstools
3. Allergy to a particular food
4. Bacterial infection e.g. Salmonella typhi-murium
5. Viral infection

Clinical features
1. Malaise
2. Nausea and vomiting
3. Abdominal colic
4. Diarrhoea

Treatment of gastroenteritis
1. The cause must be identified by stool culture and careful dietary history
2. 'Food-poisoning' due to toxins or allergy subsides spontaneously in 12–24 hours if no more of the offending food is eaten
3. Infective gastroenteritis requires careful nursing to prevent spread of the infection, and isolation and 'barrier-nursing' may be needed. Antibiotics should be given for bacterial infection
4. Severe diarrhoea causes loss of fluid and electrolytes and i.v. fluids may be needed to correct these abnormalities.
   Infective gastroenteritis is more dangerous in infants, in whom dehydration may develop rapidly

REGIONAL ILEITIS (CROHN'S DISEASE)
Patchy inflammation, often starting in the terminal ileum, with thickening of the intestinal wall and narrowing of the lumen. The cause is unknown. Although the terminal ileum is the commonest site, the disease may also involve the colon or rectum, and there may be small patches (skip lesions) in the upper ileum or jejunum.

Clinical features
1. Usually young adults
2. Malaise, weakness, weight loss, pyrexia
3. Intermittent abdominal pain with tenderness in R. iliac fossa
4. Mild or moderate diarrhoea

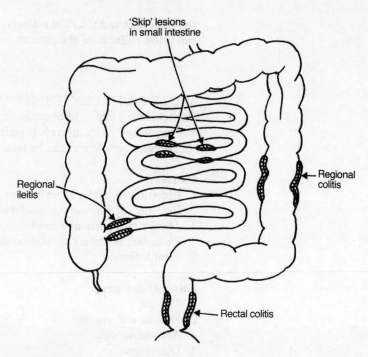

Figure 4.12
Sites affected by regional enteritis
(Crohn's disease)

Complications
1. Obstruction due to scar tissue causing strictures or adhesions
2. Perforation
3. Abscess
4. Fistula into the skin, vagina or bladder

Treatment
1. Broad spectrum antibiotics
2. Prednisone
3. Surgical resection of the affected bowel

ULCERATIVE COLITIS
In this disease the mucosa of the colon becomes thick, inflamed and
ulcerated. It is a chronic disease, but acute exacerbations are common,
and there may be periods of several months or years between attacks
when the disease is inactive. The cause is unknown, but some patients
have an obsessional personality.

Clinical features
1. Often in middle adult life (3rd or 4th decade)
2. Malaise, weakness, weight loss, pyrexia
3. Diarrhoea with blood and mucus. Often severe and chronic
4. Pain in L. iliac fossa

Complications
1. Perforation
2. Haemorrhage, dehydration, loss of electrolytes
3. May develop cancer of colon in later life

Treatment
1. Bed rest with a high-calorie, high-protein diet supplemented by vitamins and oral iron
2. Sulphasalazine ('*Salazopyrine*') or prednisone orally
3. Correction of severe anaemia or electrolyte loss by transfusion or i.v. fluids
4. Surgery for severe cases (ileostomy or colectomy)

CANCER OF THE COLON
This is a common form of cancer in elderly people.

Clinical features
1. Change in bowel habit
2. Blood or mucus in the stools
3. Intestinal obstruction
4. May be a tender mass on palpation
   The diagnosis is confirmed by a barium enema.

Treatment
Surgical resection of the affected colon.

DIVERTICULITIS
Multiple blind sacs (diverticula) form in the wall of the sigmoid colon. This is called *diverticulosis* if the sacs are asymptomatic, but *diverticulitis* if they become inflamed.

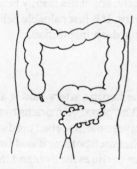

Figure 4.13
Diverticulosis. Small diverticula develop in the sigmoid colon

Clinical features
1. Usually middle-aged or elderly
2. Recurrent bouts of colicky abdominal pain
3. May be either constipation or diarrhoea
4. Tenderness in L. iliac fossa, often with a palpable mass

Complications
1. Obstruction
2. Perforation
3. Abscess
4. Fistula into bladder or vagina

Treatment
1. Analgesics
2. Broad-spectrum antibiotics e.g. tetracycline
3. Surgery for severe cases e.g. colostomy

'IRRITABLE BOWEL' SYNDROME
This common syndrome which is due to abnormal neuromuscular function of the large bowel is diagnosed by excluding other diseases by barium enema, sigmoidoscopy etc.

Clinical features
1. Colicky pain, especially after food
2. Bloating
3. Altered bowel habit
    e.g. constipation
    diarrhoea
    dry 'rabbit stools'
    mucus passed per rectum
4. Tenderness on palpation of the colon

Treatment of 'irritable bowel' syndrome
1. Increased intake of dietary roughage, e.g. wholemeal bread and bran
2. Analgesics and antispasmodics may be needed in acute attacks

The liver

ANATOMY AND PHYSIOLOGY

The liver is one of the largest organs in the body, and it lies mainly below the right diaphragm, protected by the lower ribs. It is just palpable below the rib margin in some normal people during deep inspiration.

Blood supply of the liver

The liver receives oxygenated blood from the hepatic artery, and it also receives venous blood from the portal vein. The portal vein drains blood from the small intestine and spleen and it conveys the absorbed products of digestion from the gut to the liver for further metabolism. Blood from both the hepatic artery and the portal vein thus perfuses the liver and then drains from the liver into the hepatic vein, which carries it to the inferior vena cava and thence to the heart.

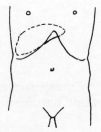
Figure 4.14
Position of normal liver

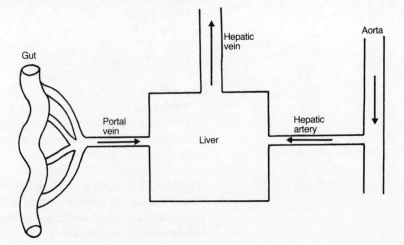
Figure 4.15
Blood supply of the liver

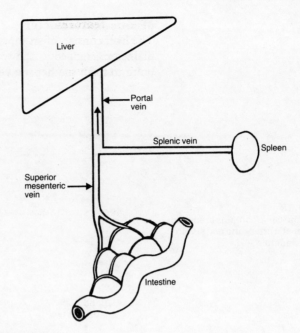

Figure 4.16
The portal drainage system. Blood from the spleen and gut drains into the liver

Drainage of bile

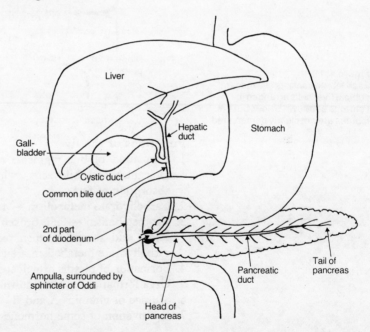

Figure 4.17
The drainage of bile and pancreatic juice

Bile formed in the liver drains into the hepatic duct, which unites with the cystic duct to form the common bile duct. The bile from the hepatic duct is stored temporarily in the gall-bladder, and is discharged down the bile duct when a fatty meal is eaten. The bile duct unites with the pancreatic duct and thus forms the ampulla of Vater which opens into the second part of the duodenum. The entry of the bile and pancreatic juices into the duodenum is controlled by the sphincter of Oddi.

Microscopic structure

The liver consists of an enormous number of lobules, each about 1 mm in diameter arranged as shown below. The central veins from each lobule unite to form the hepatic vein.

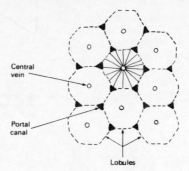

Figure 4.18
Each portal canal contains branches of the hepatic artery, the portal vein and a bile ductule

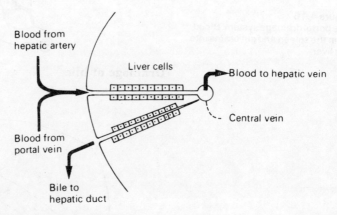

Figure 4.19
Each lobule consists of a mass of cubical liver cells arranged in columns as shown below, but the lobules are not clearly demarcated.

Functions of the liver

1. Formation of bile pigments (from the haem of the haemoglobin molecule) and bile salts (which are essential for digestion and absorption of fats)
2. Carbohydrate metabolism — formation and storage of glycogen
3. Fat metabolism — fat is broken down in the liver to glycerol and fatty acids, and these are then oxidised to produce energy. Fat and carbohydrate metabolism are closely linked
4. Formation of plasma proteins, especially albumin and clotting factors
5. Urea formation by breakdown of proteins
6. Storage of vitamins A and B_{12}
7. Inactivation of some hormones, drugs and toxins

Entero-hepatic circulation

Bile is secreted into the biliary ductules in the liver. It leaves the liver by the hepatic ducts and is stored and concentrated in the gall-bladder. When the gall-bladder contracts, bile flows along the cystic duct and common bile-duct into the duodenum. The *conjugated bilirubin* in bile is converted in the intestine into *stercobilinogen* which is the normal

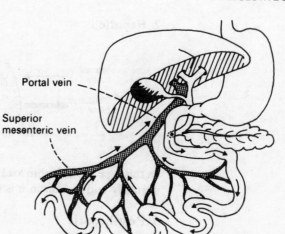

Figure 4.20

pigment in faeces. Some of this is absorbed from the intestine into the portal blood stream and returned to the liver. Most of this is re-excreted into the bile by the liver, but a small fraction escapes and is carried to the kidney and excreted in the urine as *urobilinogen*.

JAUNDICE

Yellow discolouration of the skin and sclerae of the eyes due to increased bilirubin in the blood. The normal bilirubin concentration is less than 17 μmol/litre (1 mg/100 ml).

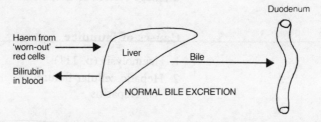

Figure 4.21

There are 3 main ways in which jaundice may be produced:

1. Pre-hepatic

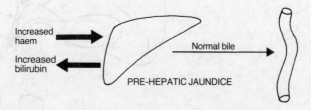

Figure 4.22

In this type there is increased breakdown of haemoglobin, usually due to haemolysis of red cells. This leads to increased formation of bilirubin in the liver, and the liver, even though it is normal, cannot excrete this increased load, so the bilirubin enters the blood stream.

2. Hepatic

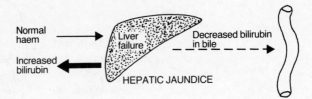

Figure 4.23

In this type the bilirubin load is normal, but the liver cells fail to function normally and so bilirubin is not excreted in adequate quantities.

3. Post-hepatic

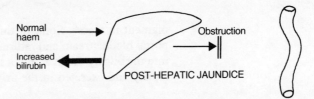

Figure 4.24

In this type the liver cells handle the bilirubin normally, but there is blockage of bile drainage (*cholestasis*). This may affect the bile ductules within the liver (*intra-hepatic cholestasis*), or it may affect the biliary drainage system after the bile has left the liver (*extra-hepatic cholestasis*).

Causes of jaundice

1. Haemolysis (p. 111)
2. Hepatic cellular failure
    (i) Hepatitis

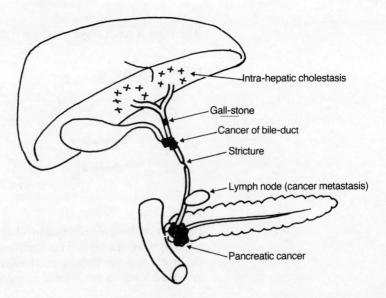

Figure 4.25
Causes of biliary obstruction (cholestasis)

(ii) Cirrhosis
(iii) Toxins e.g. carbon tetrachloride (used in dry-cleaning)
3. Obstruction of biliary tract (cholestasis). See Figure 4.25
  (i) In the lumen — gall stones
  (ii) In the wall — cholangitis
  (iii) Pressure from outside — cancer in liver, lymph nodes, pancreas, stomach

VIRAL HEPATITIS

Causes
Two strains of virus cause an identical clinical picture:
1. Virus A — transmitted in stools
  Incubation period 3–6 weeks
2. Virus B (Serum hepatitis) — transmitted by blood (transfusion, accidental inoculation etc.) which contains the Australia antigen
  Incubation period 3–6 months

Clinical features
1. Fever, malaise, anorexia
2. Jaundice develops a few days later
3. Large tender liver
4. Intra-hepatic biliary obstruction (due to cellular oedema) causes pale stools with dark urine
5. Depression and tiredness often persist after recovery

Treatment
1. Bed-rest with a high-carbohydrate, low-fat diet and avoidance of alcohol
2. In severe cases injections of pooled gamma-globulin may be given. This may also be used prophylactically

CIRRHOSIS
Fibrosis and nodular regeneration of the liver with impaired hepatic function

Causes
1. Many cases are idiopathic
2. Alcoholism
3. Following viral hepatitis

Clinical features
1. Due to hepatic failure
  (i) Jaundice and 'spider naevi' (dilated arterioles with tiny vessels radiating from them)
  (ii) Bleeding tendency (due to deficiency of prothrombin)
  (iii) Tremor, lethargy and confusion (hepatic encephalopathy)
  (iv) Weight loss and dyspepsia
  (v) Oedema

2. Due to portal hypertension:
Fibrous tissue in the liver partially obstructs the portal blood flow causing increased back-pressure and consequent dilatation in the gut veins, especially those at the lower end of the oesophagus. This causes:
   (i) Bleeding from dilated oesophageal veins (varices)
   (ii) Ascites

Treatment
1. Avoidance of alcohol
2. For oedema, a low-salt diet with spironolactone

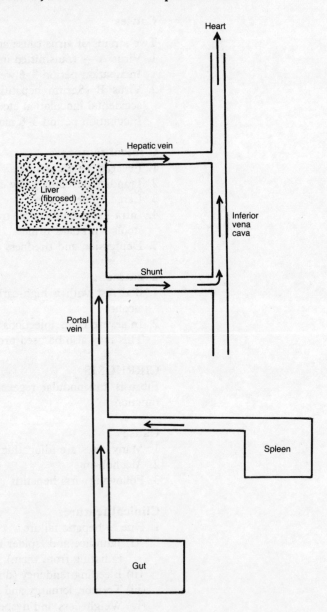

Figure 4.26
Porta-caval shunt

3. Surgery (porta-caval shunt) may be considered for the relief of portal hypertension. An anastomosis is made between the portal vein and the inferior vena cava to bypass the liver (Fig. 4.26).
4. Transfusion may be required for bleeding varices. In severe cases a special gastric tube with an inflatable balloon (Sengstaken tube) can be used to compress the varices

CHOLECYSTITIS
Inflammation of the gall-bladder, may be acute or chronic

Clinical features
1. Usually obese middle-aged patients
2. Nausea, vomiting, flatulence, fever
3. Epigastric pain, especially after fatty foods
4. Tenderness over gall-bladder, especially on deep inspiration

Treatment
1. Analgesics
2. Broad-spectrum antibiotics e.g. tetracycline

CHOLELITHIASIS
Gall-stones, often form in chronic cholecystitis

Clinical features
1. May be asymptomatic
2. Biliary colic (excruciating epigastric pain, often with vomiting)

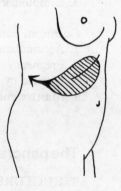

Figure 4.27
Biliary colic. Pain radiates from the R. rib margin towards the back

3. Obstructive jaundice

Complications of gall-stones
1. Cholecystitis or cholangitis
2. Perforation of gall-bladder
3. Obstruction of cystic duct or common bile duct
4. Stone in the ampulla may cause pancreatitis
5. Gall-stones predispose to malignancy of the biliary tree

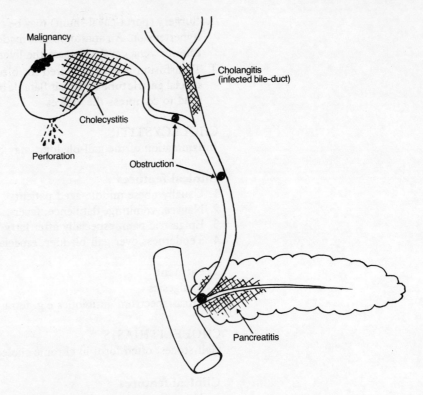

Figure 4.28
Complications of gall-stones

Treatment
1. In many cases none is needed
2. Analgesics such as morphine for biliary colic
3. Symptomatic gall-stones are usually removed surgically

Common causes of an enlarged abdomen
1. Accumulation of fat, fluid or flatus (gas)
2. Pregnancy
3. Ovarian cyst
4. Massive enlargement of liver, spleen or kidney

The pancreas

STRUCTURE AND FUNCTIONS
The pancreas lies posteriorly in the upper abdomen with its head in the loop of the duodenum and its tail near the spleen. Its duct joins with the common bile duct, and it pours its exocrine secretions into the duodenum at the ampulla of Vater (see p. 55).

Exocrine secretions
1. *Digestive enzymes*
    (i) Trypsinogen and chymotrypsinogen
    (ii) Amylase
    (iii) Lipase

2. *Sodium bicarbonate*. This neutralizes the acid secretions from the stomach

Endocrine secretions
There are also specialized groups of α and ß-cells in the pancreas which make up the islands of Langerhans. These islands secrete the following hormones directly into the blood stream, and they play a vital role in the control of carbohydrate metabolism.

1. *Glucagon* from the α cells (p. 103)
2. *Insulin* from the ß cells (p. 103)

ACUTE PANCREATITIS
Cause
Pancreatitis may follow pancreatic duct obstruction or excess of alcohol but in many cases no cause is found. It is a serious condition which can be fatal.

Clinical features
1. Severe upper abdominal pain
2. Vomiting and 'shock'

Treatment
1. Analgesics e.g. pethidine
2. Intravenous fluids as necessary for 'shock'
3. Gastric intubation and suction

CHRONIC PANCREATITIS
Follows recurrent acute pancreatitis

Clinical features
1. Malabsorption (weight loss and pale fatty stools)
2. Diabetes mellitus in some cases

Treatment
1. Low-fat diet and avoidance of alcohol
2. *Pancreatin* (enzymes) orally with meals

CARCINOMA OF THE PANCREAS
This usually occurs in the head of the pancreas and it has a very poor prognosis

Clinical features
1. Boring pain in the upper abdomen which often radiates into the back
2. Jaundice due to obstruction of the common bile duct
3. Weight loss

Treatment
Surgery, which is often only palliative

Special tests in gastroenterology

1. Radiology

(i) *Plain X-ray* of the abdomen reveals enlargement of the liver or spleen, and it shows the position of the air bubble in the fundus of the stomach. It will also show gall-stones, fluid-levels in intestinal obstruction, etc.

(ii) *Barium swallow* is used to outline the oesophagus and study its motility

(iii) *Barium meal* outlines the stomach and duodenum. A follow-through examination some hours later will outline the small intestine

(iv) *Barium enema* outlines the colon

(v) In *cholecystography* a radio-opaque dye which is excreted by the liver into the bile is given, and this outlines the gall-bladder. *Cholangiography* is a similar technique used to outline the biliary tree

2. Gastric acid production

The patient is fasted and intubated, and collections of gastric juice are obtained for analysis at 15 minute intervals. The basal and maximal acid output per hour are measured before and after stimulation with pentagastrin.

3. Jejunal biopsy

This may be obtained by persuading the patient to swallow a Crosby capsule which snips off a piece of mucosa when suction is applied.

4. Liver biopsy

This is obtained by pushing a Menghini needle into the liver whilst the patient holds his breath in deep inspiration.

5. Endoscopy

A variety of flexible fibre-optic instruments are now available for examination, photography and biopsy of the oesophagus, stomach, duodenum, jejunum and colon.

6. Proctoscopy and sigmoidoscopy

These techniques using rigid instruments allow inspection and biopsy of the rectum and sigmoid colon respectively.

FURTHER READING

Gribble H E 1977 Gastroenterological nursing. (Nurses Aids Series). Bailliere Tindall, London
Naish J M, Read A E 1974 Basic gastroenterology, 2nd edn. Wright, Bristol
Salter R H 1977 Common gastroenterological problems. Wright, Bristol

5 Nervous system

THE BRAIN

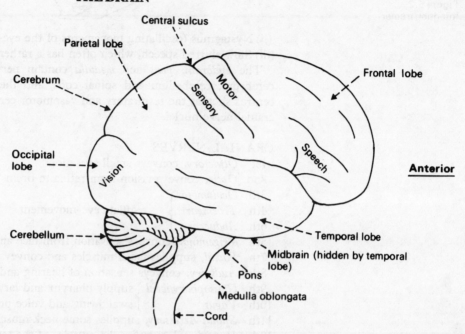

Figure 5.1

The *cerebrum* has psychic, motor and sensory functions. The two cerebral hemispheres each send and receive impulses from the opposite side of the body.

Movements are initiated by the *motor cortex*, anterior to the central sulcus.

Sensations are received by the *sensory cortex*, posterior to the central sulcus.

Vision is transmitted by the optic nerves and optic tract to the occipital lobe.

The *speech centre* is located in Broca's area in the frontal lobe of the dominant hemisphere (in a R. handed person this is the L. hemisphere).

The *cerebellum* maintains posture and regulates muscular tone and activity. Lesions of the cerebellum cause:

(i) Muscular incoordination which is most marked on voluntary movement. When the patient is asked to touch his nose with his finger, the finger oscillates wildly as it approaches the nose. This is called an intention tremor

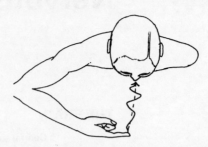

Figure 5.2
Intention tremor

(ii) Nystagmus (oscillating movements of the eye-ball)
(iii) Slow slurred speech, which often has a rather staccato quality

The *midbrain, pons* and *medulla* contain nerve tracts connecting cerebrum, cerebellum and spinal cord, and they contain important centres such as the respiratory and vasomotor centres and most of the cranial nerve nuclei.

CRANIAL NERVES

1st   *Olfactory,* conveys smell sensation
2nd   *Optic,* conveys vision from retina to brain
3rd   *Oculomotor*⎫
4th   *Trochlear* ⎬   regulate eye-movement
6th   *Abducens* ⎭
5th   *Trigeminal,* conveys sensation from face and scalp
7th   *Facial,* supplies facial muscles and conveys taste
8th   *Auditory,* conveys sensation of hearing and balance
9th   *Glossopharyngeal* ⎫ supply pharynx and larynx to regulate
10th *Vagus*   ⎭ swallowing and voice production
11th *Spinal Accessory,* supplies some neck muscles
12th *Hypoglossal,* supplies the muscles of the tongue

Common cranial nerve lesions

Optic neuritis
Degeneration or inflammation of the 2nd Cr. N. may cause misty vision and painful eye movements.

Ophthalmoplegia
Paralysis of ocular movement due to lesions of 3rd, 4th or 6th Cr. Ns may be accompanied by:
1. *Strabismus* (squint)
2. *Diplopia* (double vision)
3. *Ptosis* (drooping eyelid)

Trigeminal neuralgia
Paroxysmal attacks of excruciating pain in the distribution of the 5th Cr. N. Treatment is with the anticonvulsant drug carbamazepine, but if there is no response the nerve or its ganglion may be destroyed surgically.

Facial palsy
7th Cr. N. paralysis.

Causes
1. 'Stroke' affecting internal capsule (often with hemiplegia)
2. Bell's palsy (of unknown cause)
3. Trauma to facial nerve, or pressure on nerve e.g. from parotid tumour

THE SPINAL CORD

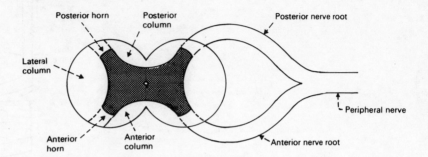

Figure 5.3
Transverse section of spinal cord

MOTOR PATHWAY
Fibres from neurones (*upper motor neurones*) in the motor cortex cross over in the medulla and descend in the lateral column of the spinal cord. These fibres end in the anterior horn and relay (synapse) with the anterior horn cells (*lower motor neurones*) which transmit impulses to the muscles via the anterior nerve root and peripheral nerve.

SENSORY PATHWAY
Sensory impulses from the peripheral nerve endings enter the spinal cord by the posterior horn. Fibres conveying position, vibration and touch travel upwards in the posterior column of the cord and cross over at the medulla. Fibres carrying pain and temperature cross over at once and travel upwards in the anterior and lateral columns. All these sensory fibres relay in the thalamus, whence impulses are conveyed to the sensory cortex.

REFLEX ACTION
Reflex action allows rapid responses e.g. withdrawal from heat. A sensory stimulus passes into the posterior horn of the spinal cord and is conveyed directly to the motor cells of the anterior horn so that a movement is made without any conscious effort by the subject. Tendon reflexes such as the knee jerks are used to test the function of the nervous system.

The knee jerk (a reflex action)
Stretching the quadriceps muscle by briskly tapping the patellar tendon initiates a reflex contraction of the muscle.

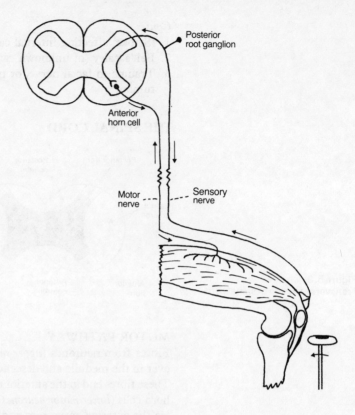

Posterior
root ganglion

Anterior
horn cell

Motor
nerve

Sensory
nerve

Figure 5.4
Reflex action

Abnormalities of movement

A. LOSS OF MOVEMENT
Paralysis is the inability to move a particular muscle
Paresis is weakness of a muscle short of complete paralysis
Monoplegia is paralysis of one limb
Hemiplegia is paralysis of the arm and leg on one side of the body
Paraplegia is paralysis of both legs

Causes of paraplegia
1. Congenital defect of brain ('spastics')
2. Trauma to spinal cord (vertebral fracture, etc.)
3. Compression of the spinal cord
    (i) Neoplasm of cord or meninges
    (ii) Abscess
    (iii) Vertebral disease (TB, osteoma, etc.)
4. Degenerative disease of the cord
    (i) Disseminated sclerosis
    (ii) Sub-acute combined degeneration due to vit. B_{12} deficiency

Spasticity and flaccidity
Lesions of the *upper motor neurones* in the brain (p. 67) or their descending fibres in the spinal cord cause *spastic paralysis*, with rigid limbs and exaggerated tendon reflexes.

Lesions of the *lower motor neurones* in the anterior horn (p. 67) or their fibres in the peripheral nerves cause *flaccid paralysis* with limp limbs and absent tendon reflexes.

B. INVOLUNTARY MOVEMENT

1. Tremor (shaking)
Causes
 (i) Parkinsonism
 (ii) Cerebellar disease
 (iii) Alcoholism
 (iv) Thyrotoxicosis

2. Spasm (involuntary contraction of a muscle)
Causes
 (i) Epilepsy
 (ii) Disseminated sclerosis
 (iii) Tetanus
In *tonic spasm* the muscle remains contracted
In *clonic spasm* the contractions are rhythmical

3. Choreiform movements
Short jerky movements seen in chorea (p. 17)

4. Athetosis
Refers to slow writhing movements, usually caused by brain damage

C. INCOORDINATION OF MOVEMENT
This is called *ataxia*.

Causes
1. Alcoholic intoxication
2. Cerebellar disease
3. Tabes dorsalis (syphilis)

The meninges and cerebrospinal fluid

The three membranes which surround and protect the brain and spinal cord are called the meninges. They are separated from each other and from the skull by potential spaces as shown in Figure 5.5

1. *Dura mater* (outer layer) is very tough
2. *Arachnoid*
3. *Pia mater* (inner layer) is fragile

The cerebrospinal fluid (c.s.f.) which bathes the brain and spinal cord is secreted by the *choroid plexuses* into the ventricles of the brain. It then passes through three small openings in the roof of the brain stem (behind the pons) into the *subarachnoid space* between the arachnoid and the pia mater. The c.s.f. then circulates over the surface of the brain and the spinal cord. It is eventually reabsorbed into the blood stream through small projections of the arachnoid mater (the *arachnoid villi*) which bulge into the venous sinus of the dura mater.

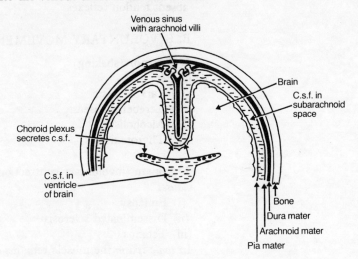

Figure 5.5
Cross-section of skull to show
circulation of cerebro-spinal fluid

A specimen of c.s.f. may be obtained by a *lumbar puncture*, in which a needle is passed between the spines of the lumbar vertebrae into the subarachnoid space.

Changes in c.s.f. may help in diagnosis:
1. Turbid or purulent c.s.f. occurs in *meningitis*. The organism may be identified by culture
2. Blood in c.s.f. occurs in *subarachnoid haemorrhage*
3. C.s.f. pressure is increased by *cerebral tumour* and *haematoma*
4. Proteins in c.s.f. may be increased in *cerebral tumour* and *disseminated sclerosis*
5. The c.s.f. Wassermann reaction is positive in *syphilis*

MENINGITIS
Inflammation of the meninges.

Causes

1. Bacterial
   (i) Meningococcal
   (ii) Tuberculous
   (iii) Pyogenic e.g. Pneumococcus, Streptococcus, Haemophilus.

2. Viral

Clinical features common to all types of meningitis
1. Fever, malaise and vomiting
2. Headache, neck stiffness and backache
3. Drowsiness, delirium, coma

Specific features
Meningococcal — a severe form, often accompanied by a purpuric rash.

Some cases develop septicaemia, with bleeding into the adrenal glands, and consequent 'shock'.

Tuberculous — often of more gradual onset and running a longer course. Many cases have permanent after-effects.

Pyogenic — may be an extension of infection from the middle ear or nasal sinuses.

Viral — tends to be relatively mild.

Complications of meningitis
1. Cranial nerve palsy
2. Focal cerebral lesions e.g. paralysis
3. Epilepsy
4. Hydrocephalus

Investigation and treatment
Lumbar puncture is required for identification of the causative organism. Bacterial sensitivities are needed to allow the appropriate antibiotic to be prescribed. In some cases this will be administered intra-thecally (i.e. into the sub-arachnoid space).

HYDROCEPHALUS
Hydrocephalus is a dilatation of the ventricles of the brain due to blockage of either the circulation or the absorption of the c.s.f.
1. Congenital hydrocephalus is due to a developmental defect in the brain. In infants the sutures between the bones are not united and so the skull enlarges to accommodate the swollen brain. The brain tissue becomes compressed and mental deficiency is common.
2. Acquired hydrocephalus is due to blockage of the c.s.f. circulation by tumour or meningitis.

Treatment of hydrocephalus
Surgical, by means of a tube inserted into the ventricles to drain off the surplus fluid.

Poliomyelitis

A viral infection which affects motor neurones in the anterior horn of the cord and the cranial nerve nuclei (p. 66). It is transmitted by droplet infection and in the faeces, but is now rare in U.K. due to vaccination.

Clinical features
1. Usually children or young adults
2. Sudden onset of an influenza-like illness, often with headache and stiff neck
3. After a few days either these symptoms subside or paralysis rapidly develops. Recovery is gradual, but permanent weakness is common and the affected muscles become atrophic
4. The brain stem may be affected with paralysis of swallowing and respiration ('bulbar polio')

Treatment
1. Strict barrier nursing and bed rest, preferably in a 'polio unit'
2. Physiotherapy, with splints and supports, is required if paralysis develops. Analgesics and sedatives may be needed
3. In bulbar polio the patient may need tracheostomy, suction of bronchial secretions, positive-pressure ventilation etc.

Prevention
Infants should be routinely immunized against polio. The vaccine is taken by mouth, often on a cube of sugar.

Neurosyphilis

About 10 per cent of patients with syphilis develop neurological disease some years after the primary infection.

There are three main types:

1. Meningo-vascular syphilis
Inflammation of the vessels to the meninges and brain causes a wide variety of CNS lesions with headache, confusion, epilepsy, localising signs etc.

2. Tabes dorsalis
Degeneration of the fibres in the posterior columns of the spinal cord may cause sharp stabbing leg pains, unsteady gait, impotence, optic atrophy, deep skin ulcers and destructive, painless arthritis (Charcot's joints).

The pupils are small, irregular and do not constrict when tested with light (Argyll Robertson pupils).

3. General paralysis of the insane (G.P.I.)
Insidious onset of dementia (intellectual deterioration) and personality change, usually in middle-aged men. Dysarthria, tremors and spastic weakness are common.

The diagnosis of these three diseases is usually confirmed by finding a positive Wasserman Reaction (W.R.) and characteristic protein changes in the cerebro-spinal fluid.

Treatment of neurosyphilis
Intramuscular penicillin, repeated until the W.R. becomes negative.

Coma

Loss of consciousness

Causes
1. Head injury
2. Epilepsy
3. Drugs e.g. alcohol, anaesthetic, hypnotics
4. Syncope (q.v.)

5. Cerebro-vascular accident (p. 75)
6. Cerebral tumour
7. CNS infection e.g. meningitis, abscess
8. Severe metabolic disturbance
    (i) Hypoglycaemia
    (ii) Diabetic ketosis
    (iii) Uraemia
    (iv) Hepatic failure
Syncope is a transient loss of consciousness due to inadequate cerebral blood-flow.

Causes of syncope
1. Vaso-vagal attack ('faint')
2. Massive bleeding
3. Stokes-Adams attack (heart-block)

Intra-cranial tumour

The terms *'intra-cranial tumour'* and *'space-occupying lesion'* are often used synonymously to include all expanding lesions inside the skull.

Causes
1. Neoplasm
2. Abscess
3. Haematoma

Common intra-cranial neoplasms
1. Glioma (malignant, arising from cerebrum)
2. Meningioma (benign, arising from meninges)
3. Secondary metastases (malignant, often from breast or bronchus)

Clinical features of intra-cranial neoplasm
1. Localizing effects, depending on the site. May be motor, sensory or psychic
2. Raised intra-cranial pressure
    (i) Headache (worse on straining) and drowsiness
    (ii) Bradycardia
    (iii) Vomiting
    (iv) Papilloedema (swelling and blurring of the optic disc)
3. Epilepsy

Epilepsy

A paroxysmal disturbance of brain function which ceases spontaneously and tends to recur.

Predisposing causes
1. Birth injury and cerebral malformation

2. Cerebral tumour
3. Trauma
4. Cerebro-vascular accident
5. Infection e.g. encephalitis or meningitis
6. Metabolic upset
   (i) Exhaustion and stress
   (ii) Anoxia
   (iii) Hypoglycaemia
   (iv) Pyrexia, especially in children
Many cases are idiopathic.

Symptoms of epilepsy
1. Loss of consciousness (partial or complete)
2. Convulsive movements
3. Sensory abnormalities
4. Autonomic disturbance, especially incontinence
5. Psychic disturbance

Types of epilepsy

1. Grand mal
The classical epileptic fit has the following stages:
  (i) *Aura* — the patient is aware a convulsion is imminent
  (ii) *Tonic* — sudden coma with generalized rigidity and absent respiration
  (iii) *Clonic* — convulsive movements, salivation and incontinence
  (iv) *Coma* — the limbs are limp with absent reflexes
  (v) *Recovery of consciousness* — may be accompanied by headache, or automatism in which the patient is unaware of his actions

2. Petit mal
A brief interruption of consciousness in which the patient may only stop what he is doing for a few seconds.

3. Focal epilepsy
Clinical features depend on the site affected. In temporal lobe epilepsy there may be bizarre movements, emotions or sensations.

4. Status epilepticus
A series of grand mal seizures wthout intervening recovery of consciousness. May be fatal if untreated.

Treatment of epilepsy
Treatment of a 'grand mal' attack:
1. Loosen the collar and maintain the airway
2. Restrain only to prevent self-injury

Prophylactic treatment
Drugs must be taken regularly to reduce the frequency of attacks
e.g. Phenobarbitone
Phenytoin } for grand mal
Ethosuximide, } for petit mal

Treatment of 'status epilepticus'
Diazepam (Valium) by slow i.v. injection, or paraldehyde by i.m. injection.

Cerebro-vascular disease

STROKE (Cerebro-vascular accident)
This is an acute cerebral catastrophe due to either infarction or bleeding into the brain.

Causes of a stroke

1. Intra-cerebral haemorrhage
Usually secondary to hypertension.

2. Cerebral infarction
This is due to thrombosis, embolism or spasm of the carotid, vertebral or cerebral vessels. Thrombosis is usually caused by atheroma of the affected vessels, and emboli usually arise from a damaged heart (e.g. mitral stenosis with atrial fibrillation, or after a myocardial infarction).

Clinical features of a stroke
1. Most patients are elderly
2. 'Transient ischaemic attacks' may cause a temporary weakness of one limb or slight difficulty with words. These are often recurrent and they presage a more severe stroke
3. Sudden onset of coma is common. This may last for only a few minutes, or for many days
4. Subsequent neurological abnormalities depend on the size and site of the lesion. Strokes commonly affect the internal capsule of the brain and they then produce hemiplegia or hemiparesis of the opposite side of the body often with dysphasia (Dysphasic patients recognize common objects but cannot think of the name for them.)
5. The prognosis varies from complete recovery to death

Treatment
1. Careful nursing is vital in the acute stages
2. Following recovery from the coma, attention must be given to rehabilitation. Physiotherapy and occupational therapy are important at this stage, but much depends on the will of the patient to recover
3. Aspirin has been shown to decrease the risk of a major stroke in patients with 'transient ischaemic attacks'

INTRA-CRANIAL HAEMORRHAGE

Since the skull acts like a closed box, haemorrhage within it increases the intra-cranial pressure, and this may cause serious complications due to compression of the brain. The clinical picture depends on the site of the haemorrhage, as follows:

1. Extra-dural haemorrhage

Figures 5.6–5.9
Types of intra-cranial haemorrhage

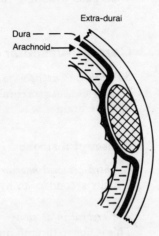

Figure 5.6

Usually a ruptured meningeal artery due to a skull fracture. Produces rapidly progressing coma due to cerebral compression. Immediate operation to relieve the pressure is required.

2. Sub-dural haematoma

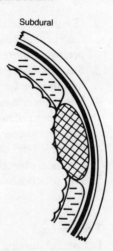

Figure 5.7

Usually follows a minor head injury in elderly patients, with blood oozing from veins into the sub-dural space. After a latent period of some days there is gradual onset of headaches, drowsiness, weakness and eventual coma.

3. Subarachnoid haemorrhage

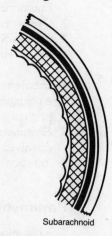

Subarachnoid

Figure 5.8

Usually a ruptured cerebral aneurysm (dilated artery). Severe headache, often occipital, followed by coma.

4. Intracerebral haemorrhage

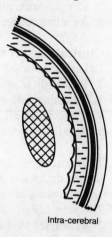

Intra-cerebral

Figure 5.9

Clinical features vary depending on the site and size of the bleed. (see Stroke, p. 75)

Migraine

The attacks are due to transient constriction, followed by dilatation, of the branches of the external carotid artery.

Clinical features
1. An 'aura' precedes the attack e.g. flashing lights, numbness or tingling
2. Paroxysmal headache, usually confined to one side of the head
3. Attacks are often accompanied by vomiting and photophobia (dislike of the light)

Factors which may precipitate migraine
1. Emotional upset or anxiety
2. Overwork
3. Certain foods e.g. chocolate
4. Fluid retention e.g. due to oral contraceptives, or premenstrually

Treatment
1. Avoidance of precipitating causes. *Sedation* or *Clonidine* may help to prevent attacks
2. *Ergotamine tartrate* should be given early in each attack, either dissolved under the tongue or as a suppository or intramuscular injection

Parkinsonism

The pathological lesion is degeneration of the *basal ganglia* of the brain. There is also depletion of a neurotransmitter called *dopamine*.

Causes
1. Idiopathic 'paralysis agitans'
2. Drugs, especially phenothiazines (e.g. chlorpromazine) in high dosage
3. As a late sequel of encephalitis

Clinical features
1. Insidious onset in elderly patients
2. Immobile face
3. Shuffling gait with characteristic posture
4. Tremor, which is most marked at rest
5. Rigidity (resistance to passive movement of a joint)

Treatment
Useful drugs include:
1. *Laevodopa,* which is converted into dopamine in the brain
2. *Amantadine (Symmetrel)*
3. *Benzhexol (Artane)*

Disseminated sclerosis

The pathological lesion is patchy demyelination (loss of white matter) of the central nervous system which may affect either the brain or the spinal cord. The cause is unknown, but there is some evidence that an abnormal immunological reaction to a viral infection may be involved.

Clinical features
1. Onset is in young adults, insidious but gradually progressive over many years. Prolonged remissions occur in the early stages
2. Spastic weakness, usually starting in legs
3. Sensory loss or paraesthesiae (tingling)
4. Diplopia (double vision) or optic neuritis (p. 66)

5. Cerebellar signs
   (i) Slow staccato speech
   (ii) Intention tremor e.g. on picking up a pin
   (iii) Nystagmus (oscillating eye movements)
6. Eventually mental changes, paraplegia with painful spasms and sphincter changes occur

Treatment
ACTH or cyanocobalamin injections may help.

Motor neurone disease

An uncommon disease of unknown cause in which progressive degeneration of the anterior horn cells in the spinal cord and the upper motor neurones in the brain causes muscle wasting and weakness.

Syringomyelia

An uncommon disease of unknown cause in which cavities develop in the spinal cord, causing progressive weakness, wasting and loss of pain and temperature sensation.

Disorders of peripheral nervous system

NEURITIS
This term refers to all types of peripheral nerve disease (degenerative, traumatic or inflammatory). The term neuropathy is more accurate.

Causes
1. Many cases are idiopathic
2. Bacterial infection e.g. leprosy, tetanus
3. Trauma e.g. compression by crutches or stretching
4. Vitamin deficiency, especially B_{12}
5. Miscellaneous metabolic upsets
   (i) Diabetes mellitus
   (ii) Chronic uraemia
   (iii) Bronchial carcinoma

Clinical features
1. Weakness or paralysis
2. Numbness or tingling, often in a 'glove and stocking' distribution
3. Trophic changes e.g. muscle wasting or skin ulcers
4. Loss of tendon reflexes
   The localization depends on which nerves are affected.
   Polyneuritis affects many nerves symmetrically and simultaneously.
If progressive and severe this can be fatal due to paralysis of respiratory muscles.

Carpal tunnel syndrome
Pain and tingling in the fingers due to compression of the median nerve at the wrist.

Causes of muscle wasting
1. Part of cachexia (generalized wasting) in severe illness such as cancer or TB
2. Atrophy due to disuse of a muscle e.g. in arthritis or limb-splinting
3. Disease of the anterior horn cells or peripheral nerves e.g. polio, motor neurone disease, peripheral neuropathy

Myasthenia gravis

A rare disease in which antibodies directed against the nerve-muscle junction cause muscles to tire very rapidly. Treatment with *neostigmine* restores the power by preventing the breakdown of acetylcholine at motor nerve-endings. Thymectomy may help to overcome the immunological abnormality which causes this disease.

Muscular dystrophy

A group of uncommon inherited diseases in which muscles degenerate with consequent loss of power. Sometimes the muscles become bulky (pseudohypertrophy) despite their weakness.

Insomnia (Inability to sleep).

COMMON CAUSES

1. Physical factors
 (i) Pain or discomfort
 (ii) Dyspnoea
 (iii) Cough
 (iv) Frequency of micturition
 (v) Flatulence
 (vi) Pruritus
 (vii) Restlessness associated with a febrile illness
(viii) Withdrawal of hypnotic drugs

2. Psychological factors
 (i) Worry or anxiety
 (ii) Excitement (may be induced by drugs or coffeee)
 (iii) Depression (especially early morning waking)
 (iv) Psychiatric illness e.g. hallucinations

3. Environmental factors
 (i) Noise
 (ii) Light

(iii) Hard bed
(iv) Cold or excess heat

Special tests in neurological disease

1. Lumbar puncture (p. 70)

2. Radiology
 (i) A plain X-ray of the skull may show fractures, and there will be displacement of the midline structures if there is a large mass in the brain. Skull X-ray is also used to assess the size of the pituitary gland
 (ii) Carotid angiogram. A radio-opaque dye is injected into the carotid artery in the neck in order to outline the vessels in the brain.
(iii) Air encephalogram. Air is injected into the c.s.f. by a lumbar puncture, and is allowed to rise into the brain where, on X-ray, it outlines the ventricles. Patients must be nursed flat after this procedure, which produces a severe headache for the next 24 hours

3. Computerized axial tomography (CAT scan)
This expensive and sophisticated equipment, which depends on the integration of multiple X-ray pictures, allows fine anatomical detail to be seen without danger or discomfort to the patient. It is particularly valuable for space-occupying lesions in the skull, such as haematoma or cerebral neoplasm, and where it is available, it has replaced the air encephalogram.

FURTHER READING

Bickerstaff E R 1978 Neurology, 3rd edn. Hodder & Stoughton, London
Kocen R S 1976 Neuromuscular system. Churchill Livingstone, Edinburgh
Matthews W B, Miller H 1979 Diseases of the nervous system, 3rd edn. Blackwell Scientific, Oxford
Purchase G 1977 Neuromedical and neurosurgical nursing. (Nurses Aids Series). Bailliere Tindall, London

6 Urinary system

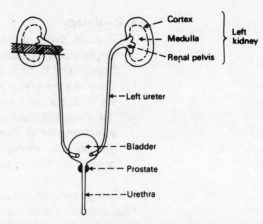

Figure 6.1
Male renal tract

Each kidney contains about one million functional units called *nephrons* (shown below). The *glomeruli* receive blood at high pressure from the afferent arterioles and the fluid filtered from the blood (*glomerular filtrate*) passes down the *tubules* to the *renal pelvis*. During its passage, the tubules selectively reabsorb various constituents (water, sodium, potassium, glucose, etc.) of the glomerular filtrate to maintain the composition of the body fluids constant.

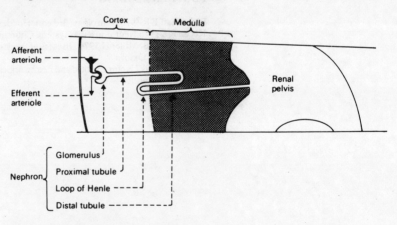

Figure 6.2
Arrangement of a nephron
(Diagrammatic view of the area shaded above in the right kidney)

FUNCTIONS OF THE KIDNEY
1. Maintenance of tissue fluids at constant composition
2. Excretion of end-products of metabolism—
   e.g. urea from protein breakdown
   uric acid from breakdown of cell nuclei
   creatinine from muscle

3. Excretion of drugs and toxins
4. Secretion of erythropoietin, which stimulates red cell production in the marrow
5. Secretion of renin, which increases blood pressure and also stimulates aldosterone secretion by the adrenal cortex (p. 102)

The kidneys excrete some substances (e.g. glucose) only when a certain concentration is exceeded in the blood. This *threshold value* varies for each substance. For glucose it is normally 10 mmol/litre (180 mg/100 ml) of blood, and glycosuria occurs only when this level is exceeded.

Urine

QUANTITY
Normally ½ to 2½ litres every 24 hours, the production rate being much greater during the day than during the night.

Causes of polyuria (increased urine production)
1. Excessive fluid intake (especially alcohol or coffee)
2. Chronic renal failure
3. Diabetes mellitus or diabetes insipidus
4. Diuretic drugs

Causes of oliguria (decreased urine production)
1. *Dehydration*
    (i) Decreased fluid intake
    (ii) Excessive sweating
    (iii) Diarrhoea, vomiting, gastric aspiration
2. *Reduced renal perfusion*
    (i) 'Shock'
    (ii) Cardiac failure
3. *Acute renal failure* (p. 87)

COLOUR
Varies, depending on concentration and on the amount of urochrome pigment. Fresh urine should be clear, but it may 'cloud' on standing. Cloudiness of fresh urine may be due to pus, bacteria or phosphates.

Causes of dark urine
1. *Blood*
    Small quantities give a smoky appearance
    Large quantities give a reddish-brown colour
2. *Bile or excessive urobilin*
3. *Ingested dyes*
    (i) Natural e.g. rhubarb, beetroot
    (ii) Synthetic e.g. coloured sweets, phenolphthalein
4. *Rare metabolic diseases* e.g. porphyria

SPECIFIC GRAVITY (S.G.)
The normal urine S.G. is 1.001 to 1.025 at room temperature
The specimen passed on rising should exceed 1.020

In renal failure the urine S.G. is constant at 1.010
Substances which increase the urine S.G.:
1. Urea or chloride
2. Glucose
3. Albumin

REACTION
The pH of normal urine is neutral or slightly acid

CHEMICAL TESTING OF URINE

Protein
A trace of protein may be found in the urine of normal subjects, but marked proteinuria is always a sign of disease. Albumin is found most commonly, but in some rare diseases globulins occur in excess in the blood and leak into the urine.

Causes of proteinuria
1. *Contamination*
   In women, with *vaginal secretion*
   In men, with *semen* or *prostatic secretion*
2. *'Postural'* (orthostatic) proteinuria
   Disappears when the patient is horizontal, and is absent from the specimen passed on rising. It does not indicate disease
3. *Renal disease*
   (i) Glomerulonephritis, especially in nephrotic syndrome
   (ii) Pyelonephritis
   (iii) Malignant hypertension
   (iv) Tuberculosis
4. *Disease of renal tract* e.g. cystitis
5. Slight albuminuria often occurs in *fevers* or in *congestive heart failure*
6. Patients with *multiple myeloma* secrete Bence-Jones protein, which coagulates on heating but redissolves on boiling

2. Blood
Haematuria (red cells in urine) is distinguished from *haemoglobinuria* (Hb without red cells) by microscopy. Haemoglobinuria is a sign of haemolysis of red cells.

Causes of haematuria
1. *Kidney lesions*
   (i) Trauma
   (ii) Glomerulonephritis, pyelonephritis or TB
   (iii) Hypernephroma
2. *Renal tract lesions*
   (i) Cystitis or bladder tumour
   (ii) Calculi from kidney or bladder
   (iii) Prostatic disease, especially carcinoma
3. *Bleeding disease or anticoagulant overdose*

Sugars
The most important is glucose (glycosuria).

Causes of glycosuria
1. Hyperglycaemia (glucose over 10 mmol/litre blood)
2. Low renal threshold (defective tubular reabsorption). In this condition glucose leaks into the urine even though the blood sugar concentration is normal, and these patients are not diabetic. It is usually of no significance.

4. Bile

Bile occurs in the urine when the patient is jaundiced, especially if this is due to biliary tract obstruction.

5. Urobilin

This is formed in the intestine during the enterohepatic circulation of bile (p. 56).

Absence of urobilin from urine indicates complete biliary tract obstruction

Excess of urobilin is due to:
  (i) Haemolysis (with excess bilirubin from Hb breakdown)
  (ii) Hepatic failure (inability of the liver to re-excrete urobilin)

6. Ketones

The ketones (acetone and two more complex molecules) are derived from the excessive breakdown of fats. If they occur in the urine the patient is said to be ketotic.

Causes of ketosis
1. Starvation
2. Uncontrolled diabetes mellitus
3. Prolonged vomiting

Micturition

The emptying of the bladder is normally controlled by the nervous system. A full bladder (300–400 ml) stimulates impulses along the afferent fibres to the sacral part of the spinal cord. The micturition reflex is normally inhibited by the brain until a convenient time, when efferent impulses from the spinal cord contract the bladder musculature and simultaneously the urethral sphincter muscle relaxes.

DISORDERS OF MICTURITION

A. Incontinence (absence of voluntary control)

Causes
1. Infancy
2. Nocturnal enuresis (bed-wetting during sleep)
3. Coma or epileptic fit
4. Spinal cord injury or disease (e.g. tumour)
5. 'Stress incontinence', due to weakness of the pelvic floor muscles or urethral sphincter. Any rise of intra-abdominal pressure (e.g. laughing, coughing, sneezing) causes a leak of urine

6. Confusion, especially in the elderly
7. Cystitis may occasionally cause incontinence

Treatment
1. In bed-ridden patients careful nursing is vital to prevent maceration of the skin and 'pressure sores'
2. The underlying cause must be treated

B. Retention of urine

Common causes in the male
1. Post-operative
2. Prostatic enlargement
3. Urethral stricture

Common causes in the female
1. Trauma of labour
2. Pressure on bladder neck from uterus enlarged by pregnancy or a fibroid
   Other causes in both sexes include:
   (i) Stones (from kidney or bladder)
   (ii) Neoplasm of bladder
   (iii) Clot (bleeding from kidney or bladder)
   (iv) Spinal cord injury or disease (e.g. disseminated sclerosis)
   It is most important to distinguish *urine retention* from *anuria* (p. 87). This can be done by palpating and percussing the supra-pubic area to see whether the bladder is distended.

'Retention with overflow'. As the bladder becomes hugely distended the pressure forces open the sphincter and small quantities of urine leak out periodically. The distended bladder is easily felt as a firm round mass above the pubis.

C. Frequency of micturition

Causes
1. *Polyuria* (p. 83)
2. *'Irritation' of the bladder or urethra*
   (i) Cystitis
   (ii) Calculus
   (iii) Pressure from pregnancy or pelvic tumour
3. *Anxiety* (e.g. before interview or examination)

D. Dysuria (painful micturition)

Causes
1. Pyelonephritis
2. Cystitis
3. Urethritis

E. Hesitancy, poor stream and dribbling

In *hesitancy* the urine flow is delayed after voluntary relaxation of the sphincter.

A *poor stream,* due to partial urethral obstruction, prolongs micturition.

Dribbling implies continuing leakage of drops of urine after the end of micturition.

These three symptoms are characteristic of prostatic hypertrophy.

Renal failure

This may be acute or chronic.

In *acute* failure the kidneys may produce little urine (*oliguria*) or no urine (*anuria*).

In *chronic* failure they may fail to respond to antidiuretic hormone (p. 97) leading to the constant production of large quantities of dilute urine of fixed specific gravity (usually 1.010).

Metabolic effects of renal failure

1. *Uraemia* [blood urea exceeding 5.5 mmol/litre (40 mg/100 ml)] due to accumulation of protein metabolites
2. *Hyperkalaemia* due to potassium retention
3. *Hyponatraemia* due to loss of sodium in urine
4. *Hypoproteinaemia* due to loss of albumin in urine
5. *Hypocalcaemia* due to loss of calcium in urine
6. *Acidosis* (decreased blood pH)

'URAEMIA'

This term is often used to refer to the overall clinical picture of advanced renal failure.

Clinical features of 'uraemia'

1. Loss of energy, drowsiness, confusion
2. Anorexia, nausea, vomiting, hiccups
3. Pruritis, pallor and 'earthy' pigmentation
4. 'Air hunger' (Kussmaul breathing) due to acidosis (p. 28)
5. Cardiac arrhythmia or cardiac arrest, due to hyperkalaemia
6. Osteomalacia or secondary hyperparathyroidism, due to hypocalcaemia

Treatment of 'uraemia'

This will vary according to whether the renal failure is acute (see p. 88) or chronic (see p. 89).

ACUTE RENAL FAILURE

Causes

1. 'Shock'
   (i) Blood loss or fluid loss
   (ii) Hypotension e.g. myocardial infarction
   (iii) Septicaemia
   (iv) Obstetric disasters e.g. abortion or ante-partum haemorrhage
2. Acute glomerulonephritis or pyelonephritis
3. Severe crush injuries

Clinical features
1. Oliguria (urine output below 500 ml/24 hours)
2. 'Uraemia' (see p. 87)

Treatment
1. Correction of fluid and electrolyte loss. For an adult the fluid intake is about 500 ml plus the volume of urine passed in the previous 24 hours. It is usually given as a concentrated glucose solution to supply calories to minimize tissue breakdown
2. An anabolic steroid to minimize tissue breakdown
3. Resonium A (binds potassium in the intestine) to lower plasma potassium
4. If necessary, peritoneal dialysis or haemodialysis

If recovery of renal function occurs the patient enters a *diuretic phase*, with large volumes of dilute urine. Large amounts of water, sodium and potassium are lost and may need to be replaced.

Glomerulonephritis

This term is applied to diffuse inflammatory disease affecting the glomeruli. It is probably due to complex immunological reactions to a variety of antigenic stimuli, including infection with ß-haemolytic streptococci or viruses. It is classified by the histological appearance of a renal biopsy specimen:
1. **Minimal change** — changes seen only on electron microscopy
2. **Membranous —** diffuse thickening of the glomerular capillary walls
3. **Proliferative —** increased number of cells in all glomeruli
4. **Focal —** proliferative changes seen in only some parts of some glomeruli

There are two main clinical types of glomerulonephritis:
1. *Acute nephritis*
2. *Nephrotic syndrome*
Either can develop hypertension or progress to chronic renal failure, and many intermediate types occur

ACUTE NEPHRITIS

Clinical features
1. Often youngsters with a history of Streptococcal tonsillitis one to three weeks previously
2. Sudden onset of headache, pyrexia, vomiting, loin pain
3. Scanty urine, with albuminuria and a smoky appearance due to haematuria
4. Moderate oedema, often periorbital, and worse in the morning

Prognosis
Most cases recover completely in a few weeks, but some die of acute renal failure or develop progressive chronic renal failure

Treatment
1. Bed rest
2. Penicillin for a few days to eradicate Streptococci

3. High calorie diet, with restriction of protein, fluid and salt until the diuretic phase occurs

NEPHROTIC SYNDROME

This is characterized by:
1. Heavy proteinuria
2. Low plasma proteins
3. Massive oedema

Glomerulonephritis is by far the commonest cause of the nephrotic syndrome but it is occasionally secondary to other disease e.g. diabetes.

Clinical features

1. Insidious onset of oedema, with a pale puffy face. The oedema becomes generalized, often with ascites or pleural effusion
2. Increased susceptibility to infections

Prognosis

Variable, but oedema may persist for months or years. Many patients ultimately develop renal failure.

Treatment

1. High protein diet with restriction of salt
2. Diuretics (p. 145)
3. Prednisone or immunosuppressive drugs such as azathioprine
4. Paracentesis (drainage) of ascites or pleural effusion

CHRONIC RENAL FAILURE

Common causes

1. Glomerulonephritis
2. Pyelonephritis
3. Malignant hypertension
4. Urinary tract obstruction e.g. stones or prostatic enlargement

Clinical features

1. *Nocturia* (increased nocturnal urine production) is an early symptom, followed eventually by *polyuria*
2. 'Uraemia' develops insidiously (p. 87)

Treatment

1. Fluid intake should be at least 3 litres daily, because in chronic renal failure the excretion of urea etc., is proportional to the urinary flow. Salt supplements may be needed
2. Low protein diet (e.g. 40 g daily). In more advanced cases the Giovanetti diet is used, with vitamin supplements
3. Blood transfusion may be needed for severe anaemia
4. Hypertension should be controlled (p. 13)
5. Dialysis with artificial kidney or renal transplant should be considered

Urinary tract infection

The urinary tract consists of the renal pelvis, ureter, bladder and urethra.

CYSTITIS
Inflammation of the bladder, usually due to bacterial infection

Common bacterial causes
1. *Escherischia coli*
2. *Streptococcus faecalis*
3. *Proteus vulgaris*
4. *Pseudomonas pyocyaneus*

It predominantly affects women, since the short female urethra readily allows bacteria to spread from the perineum to the bladder.

Infection can also descend from an infected kidney, and conversely infection of the lower urinary tract is often followed by acute pyelonephritis.

Other predisposing causes:
 (i) Retention of urine
(ii) Calculi
(iii) Bladder diverticula or cancer

Clinical features
1. Frequency of micturition, with dysuria
2. Cloudy urine with offensive odour
3. May be rigors, pyrexia and supra-pubic tenderness

Treatment (see p. 149)

ACUTE PYELONEPHRITIS
Infection of the renal pelvis, often also involving the kidney tissue

Predisposing causes
1. Lower urinary tract infection, especially if accompanied by urinary stasis (e.g. pregnancy, prostatic hypertrophy, paraplegia etc.)
2. Reflux of urine up the ureters due to urethral or ureteric dysfunction
3. Pre-existing renal disease
4. Pre-existing systemic disease e.g. diabetes mellitus

Clinical features
1. Sudden onset of fever, rigors and malaise
2. Pain and tenderness in one or both loins
3. Frequency, dysuria and cloudy offensive urine

Treatment of cystitis and acute pyelonephritis
1. High fluid intake
2. Antibacterial drugs according to bacterial sensitivity e.g. sulphonamides, cotrimoxazole, ampicillin, nalidixic acid or nitrofurantoin
3. Sodium bicarbonate to keep the urine alkaline

Follow-up urine cultures are essential to ensure the infection is eradicated. The underlying cause should be treated if possible since recurrent infection can lead to fatal chronic pyelonephritis.

CHRONIC PYELONEPHRITIS
The pathogenesis is poorly understood but recurrent infection seems to produce small scarred kidneys and eventual renal failure. In some cases the onset is insidious with sterile urine and no history of urinary tract infection.

Clinical features
1. May resemble acute pyelonephritis
2. Asymptomatic proteinuria for years, followed by progressive renal failure

Treatment
1. Prolonged treatment (several months) with appropriate anti-bacterial drugs according to sensitivity
2. Treatment of renal failure (pp. 88, 89)
Renal failure is often precipitated by an exacerbation of the infection or an electrolyte disturbance (e.g. from prolonged vomiting).

CALCULI
Calculi (stones) may form either in the kidney or the bladder, and they usually consist of calcium salts, phosphates, urates or mixtures.
Factors which predispose to stone formation:
1. Excess calcium in the urine e.g. hyperparathyroidism
2. Excess urates in the urine e.g. gout
3. Urinary tract infections e.g. cystitis
4. Stasis of urine e.g. prostatic enlargement

Clinical features
1. A stone may produce no symptoms if it remains in the kidney
2. A stone entering the ureter produces *renal colic*.

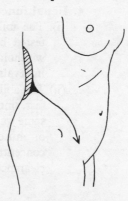

Figure 6.3
Renal colic. Pain radiates from the loin towards the genitalia

In this condition there is paroxysmal severe pain in the loin radiating into the abdomen and groin, often with haematuria. The patient is often restless, sweating and vomiting.
3. A stone in the bladder may cause dysuria and frequency

4. Small stones may pass uneventfully through the urethra. Larger ones may lodge and cause retention of urine

Treatment
1. For renal colic, morphine or pethidine may be needed
2. Stones may pass naturally but failing this, operative removal may be required
3. Correction of predisposing cause

Special tests in urinary tract disease

1. Urine examination
(i) Chemical (p. 84)
(ii) Microscopic and bacteriological. This may reveal the presence in the urine of white cells, red cells, 'casts' of the renal tubules, or bacteria

2. Radiology
Plain X-rays of the kidney yield only limited information, but in pyelonephritis they may show a small scarred kidney, and some renal calculi are radio-opaque.

Intravenous pyelogram (IVP) A radio-opaque dye which is excreted by the kidney is injected i.v., and X-ray pictures are taken at intervals to outline the kidney, its pelvis and the ureters and bladder. In *retrograde pyelography* a cystoscope is passed, and the dye is injected up the ureters from below.

3. Cystoscopy
An illuminated tube, the cystoscope, is passed through the urethra into the bladder. The bladder walls can be inspected and biopsied, and the ureteric opening can be seen and, if necessary, catheterized to allow urine to be collected from one kidney.

4. Renal function tests
(i) The ability of the kidney to excrete or to conserve water can be tested by giving either a large drink of water (1 litre) or by withholding fluids, and then collecting the urine at regular intervals and measuring its specific gravity
(ii) The ability to excrete urea is assessed by the creatinine clearance test, since urea and creatinine are handled by the glomeruli in the same way. The clearance of creatinine, which is a normal product of muscle metabolism, may be calculated by measuring its concentration in plasma and in a 24 hour urine specimen. The clearance is reduced in renal failure.

FURTHER READING

Jameson R M 1976 Management of the urological patient. Churchill Livingstone, Edinburgh
Mitchell J P 1980 Urology for nurses, 3rd edn. Wright, Bristol
Uldall R 1977 Renal nursing, 2nd end. Blackwell Scientific, Oxford

7 Reproduction

Female reproductive system

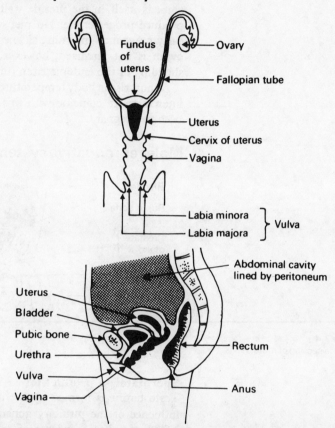

Figure 7.1
Diagram of female genitalia

Fundus of uterus

Ovary

Fallopian tube

Uterus

Cervix of uterus

Vagina

Labia minora
Labia majora } Vulva

Figure 7.2
Mid-line section of female pelvis

Abdominal cavity lined by peritoneum

Uterus
Bladder
Pubic bone
Urethra
Vulva
Vagina

Rectum

Anus

The menstrual cycle, ovulation and conception

Menstruation, which starts at puberty, is controlled by the cyclical release of *gonadotrophins* (LH and FSH) from the anterior pituitary (p. 97). The menstrual flow lasts 3 to 5 days, and recurs at regular intervals of about 28 days until the menopause at age 40 to 50.

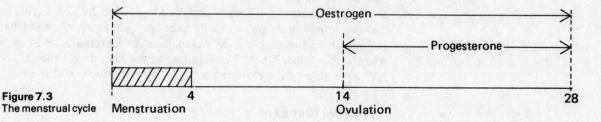

Figure 7.3
The menstrual cycle

Oestrogen

Progesterone

Menstruation   Ovulation

4   14   28

The ovaries produce oestrogen throughout the cycle. Every month in midcycle (day 14) one of the two ovaries produces an ovum from a *follicle*. The follicle matures during the first half of the cycle under the influence of follicle-stimulating hormone (FSH) from the pituitary, and on day 14 the mature ovum is expelled and enters the Fallopian tube (oviduct). The follicle is then converted into a *corpus luteum* which secretes progesterone to prevent further ovulation. If the ovum is fertilized by a sperm it embeds itself in the uterine wall and the corpus luteum continues to produce progesterone. No menstruation occurs and the symptoms of early pregnancy (morning sickness, breast tingling etc.) develop. If the ovum is not fertilized, however, the corpus luteum degenerates and shedding of the endometrium (uterine lining) starts on day 28.

A short rise in body temperature occurs shortly after ovulation. Timing intercourse to coincide with this rise may, therefore, help a woman to become pregnant.

Male reproductive system

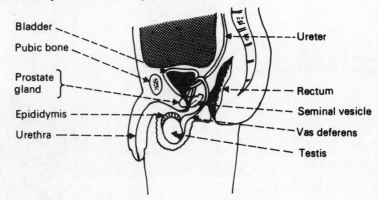

Figure 7.4
Mid-line section of male pelvis

Spermatazoa production

Testosterone is formed by the interstitial cells of the testis under the influence of the pituitary gonadotrophins. Sperms are formed in the coiled *seminiferous tubules* of the testis, and are then stored in their millions in the vas deferens until ejaculation of *semen* occurs.

Formation of sperms starts at puberty and continues until old age. If sexual intercourse or masturbation does not occur, spontaneous discharge of semen may occur in the sleep ('wet dream').

Sex of the fetus

During the formation of sperms and ova a 'reduction division' occurs so that the chromosomes are halved. Females have XX chromosomes so that each ovum carries only one X. Males have XY chromosomes so each sperm carries either X or Y. The resulting fetus is, therefore, either XX or XY depending on the chromosome carried by the successful sperm.

Venereal diseases

Diseases transmitted by sexual intercourse.

GONORRHOEA
Infection by the gonococcus (*Neisseria gonorrhoea*)
Incubation period 3 to 10 days

Clinical features

Male
1. Purulent urethral discharge
2. Scalding on micturition
3. Tender lymph nodes in the groin

Female
1. May be no symptoms
2. Scalding on micturition
3. Vaginal discharge

Complications

Male
1. Urethral stricture
2. Orchitis (inflammation of the testis)

Female
1. Salpingitis (inflammation of the Fallopian tubes)
2. Infertility (due to blocked Fallopian tubes)
Arthritis and rash may occur in either sex.
   Gonorrhoea in pregnancy can cause *ophthalmia neonatorum* (infection of the baby's eyes) due to gonococcal infection from the birth canal.

Treatment of gonorrhoea
A single large dose of i.m. penicillin will cure most cases, but resistant gonococci may need another antibiotic such as kanamycin.

SYPHILIS
Infection by a spirochaete (*Treponema pallidum*)
Incubation period 3 to 5 weeks

Clinical features of acquired syphilis
In the adult there are three stages:

1. *Primary syphilis*
The site of infection (e.g. penis, vulva, cervix, rectum, nipple or mouth) develops a hard painless 1 cm ulcer called a *chancre*, and the regional lymph nodes enlarge.

2. *Secondary syphilis*
This develops about 6 weeks later, and can persist for up to 2 years:
 (i) Tiredness, malaise, fever, sore throat, headache
 (ii) Slight generalized lymphadenopathy
(iii) A non-irritable maculo-papular rash, often involving palms and soles
(iv) Condylomata lata (moist warty papules) around the genitalia or anus
 (v) Patchy alopecia

3. *Tertiary syphilis*
This develops 2 to 20 years from the onset, after a latent period free from symptoms. It may take several forms:
  (i) Cardiovascular syphilis, e.g. aortitis; aortic incompetence; aortic aneurysm
  (ii) Neurosyphilis (p. 72)
  (iii) *Gumma* (granulomatous inflammation) of skin, bone, liver or testis

Congenital syphilis
Infection of the baby via the placenta is now rare in the U.K. due to routine *Wasserman Reaction* (W.R.) blood tests in ante-natal clinics. Congenital syphilis can cause abortion, still-birth, deafness, blindness, rash, deformed bones and teeth, etc.

Diagnosis of syphilis
In primary syphilis the spirochaete can be found in the chancre. In secondary and tertiary syphilis the W.R. is positive.

Treatment
Penicillin injections for 10 days. The course may need to be repeated until the W.R. becomes negative.

TRICHOMONAS VAGINALIS
This is a protozoon which causes *vaginal discharge* and *irritation* in women and *balanitis* (inflammation of the foreskin) in men. Treatment is with metronidazole (Flagyl) orally, which should also be given to the sexual partner.

NON-SPECIFIC URETHRITIS
The cause is unknown, but it may be due to a virus or mycoplasma.

Clinical features
1. Frequency and scalding on micturition
2. Urethral discharge

Complications
Some patients develop *Reiter's syndrome*, with arthritis, conjunctivitis and a rash

Treatment
Tetracyclines may help

FURTHER READING

Catterall R D 1979 Venereology and genito-urinary medicine: a textbook of the sexually transmitted diseases, 2nd edn. Hodder & Stoughton, London
Schofield C B S 1979 Sexually transmitted diseases, 3rd edn. Churchill Livingstone, Edinburgh
Thomson J A 1976 Introduction to clinical endocrinology. Churchill Livingstone, Edinburgh

8 Endocrinology

Exocrine glands produce an external secretion via a duct e.g. sweat, sebaceous, lacrimal and mammary glands.

Endocrine glands secrete hormones ('chemical messengers') into the blood.

The pituitary gland

The pituitary lies in the pituitary fossa, just above and behind the nasal cavity. The *hypothalamus* regulates pituitary activity by a series of '*releasing*' and '*inhibiting*' factors which pass along small blood vessels (the portal tract) linking the hypothalamus to the pituitary. The pituitary hormones control most of the other endocrine glands, and their hormones, in turn, have a '*negative feed-back*' effect on the hypothalamus.

The **anterior** pituitary secretes the following hormones:
1. *Thyrotrophin* (also called thyroid-stimulating hormone, TSH) stimulates the thyroid
2. *Corticotrophin* (ACTH) stimulates the adrenal cortex
3. *Somatotrophin* (Human growth hormone, HGH) stimulates growth
4. *Melanocyte stimulating hormone* (MSH) stimulates pigmentation
5. *Gonadotrophins* stimulate the gonads
   (i) Follicle-stimulating hormone (FSH) in the female, and interstitial cell-stimulating hormone (ICSH) in the male
   (ii) Luteinizing hormone (LH)
6. *Somatomammotrophin* (prolactin, luteotrophin) stimulates the mammary glands

The **posterior** pituitary secretes the following hormones:
1. *Antidiuretic hormone* (ADH) stimulates water reabsorption by the renal tubules
2. *Oxytocin* initiates labour and enhances uterine contractions

HYPERPITUITARISM
Pituitary over-activity, usually due to a pituitary adenoma (benign tumour).

Excessive HGH secretion during childhood causes *gigantism* with an eventual height of 7 or 8 feet.

Excessive HGH during adult life causes *acromegaly* with large hands and feet, characteristic coarse features, jutting jaw and thick greasy skin.

The pressure of a pituitary adenoma on the optic chiasma (crossing of the optic nerves) may cause loss of vision.

HYPOPITUITARISM
Pituitary under-activity

Causes

1. Pituitary necrosis following severe haemorrhage during pregnancy or childbirth
2. Non-secreting adenoma
3. Pituitary destruction by surgery or irradiation

Clinical features

In *children*, dwarfism and failure of sexual maturation

In *adults*:

1. Loss of body hair, loss of libido and cessation of menstruation
2. Pale thin skin
3. Hypothyroidism (p. 99)
4. Hypoadrenalism (p. 103)

Diabetes insipidus

Lack of ADH secretion by the posterior pituitary leads to the production of large volumes of dilute urine and frequent thirst.

This may respond to regular inhalation of a snuff prepared from the posterior pituitary. Paradoxically, some cases also respond to a diuretic, chlorothiazide.

The thyroid gland

The thyroid gland lies just below the thyroid cartilage, and the 4 small parathyroid glands are behind the thyroid.

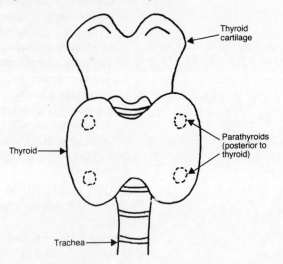

Figure 8.1
Thyroid and parathyroid glands

The thyroid, which consists of two lobes connected by an isthmus, secretes two hormones:

1. *Thyroxine* stimulates tissue metabolism. It increases oxygen consumption and heat production

   Over-production of thyroxine causes hyperthyroidism

   Under-production of thyroxine causes hypothyroidism

   A person producing the normal amount of thyroxine is said to be *euthyroid*

2. *Calcitonin* increases calcium deposition in bone, but its importance is uncertain.

GOITRE

A thyroid enlargement which may or may not secrete excess thyroxine
A 'toxic' goitre is overactive and causes thyrotoxicosis
With a 'non-toxic' goitre the patient remains euthyroid, but the goitre may press on the trachea or oesophagus

Causes of a 'non-toxic' goitre
1. A temporary goitre is common at puberty and during pregnancy
2. Iodine deficiency
3. Many cases are idiopathic

HYPERTHYROIDISM (THYROTOXICOSIS)
Hyperthyroidism is occasionally due to overproduction of TSH by the pituitary, but more commonly the thyroid becomes overactive even with normal levels of TSH. The cause in these patients is obscure, but it may sometimes be due to stimulation by an abnormal circulating antibody called *long-acting thyroid stimulator* (LATS).

Clinical features
1. Goitre which may be diffuse or nodular
2. Fine tremor
3. Warm moist skin and intolerance of heat
4. Weight loss, increased appetite and diarrhoea
5. Rapid bounding pulse
6. Tiredness and nervousness
7. May be exophthalmos (protruding eyeballs)

Complications
1. Atrial fibrillation
2. Heart failure

Treatment
1. Antithyroid drugs e.g. thiouracil, carbimazole. The dose must be carefully adjusted or the patient may become hypothyroid. Rashes and agranulocytosis may also develop.
2. Partial thyroidectomy, especially for large goitres. The surgeon must be careful to preserve the parathyroids.
3. Radio-iodine is used in older patients. The response is slow, and many patients then develop myxoedema in later years.

HYPOTHYROIDISM (MYXOEDEMA)

Causes

Primary (Thyroid gland failure)
1. Autoimmune thyroiditis
2. Iatrogenic:
    (i) Surgery (after thyroidectomy)

    (ii) Irradiation
    (iii) Excessive antithyroid medication
3. Cretinism (dwarfism and mental deficiency due to congenital hypothyroidism) is due to maternal iodine deficiency

Secondary
TSH deficiency due to pituitary failure

Clinical features
1. Mental and physical sluggishness
2. Dry rough skin with sparse hair and periorbital puffiness
3. Croaking voice and slow speech
4. Cold intolerance
5. Weight gain, constipation
6. Bradycardia (slow pulse)

Treatment
Maintenance with 0.3 mg l-thyroxine daily. A much lower dose may be advisable initially to avoid precipitating cardiac failure.

The parathyroids

The pea-sized glands, embedded in the posterior aspect of the thyroid, which secrete *parathormone*.

Action of parathormone on calcium metabolism
There is an inverse relationship between the levels of calcium and phosphate in the blood, so that as phosphate falls, calcium increases.
    Parathormone acts on the renal tubules to increase the loss of phosphate in the urine. This lowers the phosphate level in the blood and to compensate for this the blood calcium is increased by increasing calcium mobilization from the bones. The net result of parathormone is to increase the serum calcium at the expense of the bones.

HYPERPARATHYROIDISM
Parathormone excess

Causes
1. Parathyroid adenoma or hyperplasia (overactivity)
2. Parathyroid overactivity secondary to chronic renal failure or osteomalacia

Clinical features
1. Anorexia and constipation due to hypercalcaemia (increased blood calcium)
2. Renal stone due to increased urinary calcium and phosphate excretion
3. Bone pain, deformity and fractures due to thinning of bones

Treatment
Surgical: partial parathyroidectomy or removal of the adenoma

HYPOPARATHYROIDISM
Parathormone deficiency

Usually follows accidental removal of the parathyroids during thyroidectomy. The resulting hypocalcaemia causes *tetany*.

Clinical features
1. Paraesthesiae ('pins and needles') of digits
2. Muscle spasm of hands and feet. The spasm is increased by applying a tourniquet to the limb (Trousseau's sign)
3. Increased tendon reflexes
4. May be convulsions, especially in children

Tetany may also result from *acidosis* due to the depletion of carbon dioxide in the blood by over-breathing.

Treatment
Tetany due to hypocalcaemia is abolished by the slow intravenous injection of calcium gluconate.

Thereafter, dietary supplements of calcium and vitamin D.

The adrenal glands

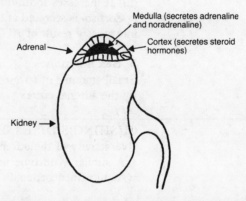

Figure 8.2
An adrenal gland

These two glands lie immediately above the kidneys. Each gland has two parts:
1. The central *medulla* secretes the catecholamines, *noradrenaline* and *adrenaline*
2. The outer *cortex* secretes a variety of *steroid* hormones

SECRETIONS FROM THE MEDULLA
Noradrenaline is the chemical transmitter at sympathetic nerve endings

It thus causes vasoconstriction and raises the blood pressure

Adrenaline prepares the body for physical activity — the 'fight, fright or flight' reaction. Its actions include:
1. Dilatation of pupils and bronchioles
2. Constriction of sphincters and inhibition of peristalsis
3. Acceleration of heart rate and increase in cardiac contractile force
4. Breakdown of liver glycogen with a consequent rise in blood glucose

SECRETIONS FROM THE CORTEX

1. Mineralocorticoids

Aldosterone conserves body sodium by stimulating sodium reabsorption in the renal tubules. The blood volume is probably regulated by the complicated *renin-angiotensin* system as follows:

A fall in blood volume produces a fall in blood pressure. This stimulates the kidneys to secrete renin which converts a circulating plasma protein called angiotensinogen into angiotensin. Angiotensin stimulates the release of aldosterone from the adrenals, which produces sodium retention, and this results in an increase in the osmotic pressure of the tissue fluids. This releases ADH from the posterior pituitary and the diminution in urine flow results in water retention and an increased blood volume.

2. Glucocorticoids

Cortisol (hydrocortisone) has several effects:

 (i) It is anti-inflammatory and anti-allergic
 (ii) It increases protein breakdown and decreases the use of carbohydrates
(iii) It increases sodium and water retention

Cortisol is secreted at times of stress, e.g. during infections or after an injury, as a result of ACTH release from the pituitary.

3. Sex hormones

Small amounts of *testosterone, oestrogen* and *progesterone* are synthesized by the adrenal cortex.

CUSHING'S DISEASE

Overactivity of the adrenal cortex

A similar syndrome may be produced by prolonged treatment with systemic glucocorticoids (i.e. steroids such as prednisone)

Causes

1. Adrenal hyperplasia secondary to pituitary overactivity
2. Adenoma or rarely adrenal carcinoma

Clinical features

1. Obesity of trunk and face, often with plethoric complexion and hirsutism
2. Hypertension
3. Striae (stretch-marks), easy bruising and pigmentation
4. Muscle weakness and bone thinning, often with vertebral collapse

Treatment

Surgical. Usually adrenalectomy but some cases secondary to pituitary disease require hypophysectomy.

Adrenal tumours which secrete excess sex hormones can cause precocious puberty in children or virilization in women

PHAEOCHROMOCYTOMA

Overactivity of the adrenal medulla. This is a very rare disease which causes paroxysmal hypertension due to the intermittent release of adrenaline and noradrenaline into the circulation.

HYPOADRENALISM

Underactivity of the adrenal gland. Both the cortex and the medulla may be affected, but symptoms are mainly due to the deficiency of the cortical hormones.

Causes

1. Addison's disease (auto-immune adrenalitis)
2. Adrenal tuberculosis
3. Prolonged glucocorticoid therapy (e.g. prednisone) causes 'adrenal suppression'

Clinical features

1. Debility and tiredness
2. Nausea and vomiting
3. Pigmentation affecting skin and oral mucosa
4. Low blood pressure
5. Adrenal 'crisis' may occur, with vomiting and severe shock due to circulatory collapse. This may be fatal unless intravenous hydrocortisone is speedily given.

Treatment

Daily hormone replacement with cortisone, with fludrocortisone to increase sodium retention.

The pancreas

In addition to its exocrine secretions (p. 40), the pancreas produces two hormones:

1. *Glucagon,* produced by the α-cells, increases blood glucose by increasing the breakdown of liver glycogen
2. *Insulin,* produced by the ß-cells, decreases blood glucose by inhibiting glycogen breakdown and facilitating the entry of glucose into tissue cells.

DIABETES MELLITUS

A metabolic disorder in which the tissues fail to use glucose, which results in *hyperglycaemia* (increased blood sugar) and *glycosuria* (excretion of sugar in the urine).

Since the tissues cannot use glucose to provide energy, fats are broken down at an increased rate and this causes *ketosis* (excessive formation of ketones, p. 85).

Causes

1. Usually idiopathic. Predisposing factors include obesity (in middle-aged people) and a family history of diabetes. In young patients an

auto-immune, mechanism may operate, and these cases of 'juvenile diabetes' are often very severe.

2. Occasionally secondary to:
   (i) Other disease e.g. pancreatitis, acromegaly
   (ii) Drugs e.g. prednisone, diuretics

Clinical features

1. Weight loss and weakness due to inability to use glucose
2. Polyuria (increased urine production) due to the osmotic effect of glucose in urine
3. Thirst due to the polyuria

Complications

1. *Ocular*
   (i) Cataract (opacity in the lens)
   (ii) Retinopathy (haemorrhage, exudate, retinal detachment, etc.)
2. *Neurological*
   Numbness and paraesthesiae, especially in the lower limbs
3. *Renal*
   Pyelonephritis and glomerulonephritis
4. *Vascular*
   Occlusion of vessels may cause gangrene of feet, myocardial infarction or 'stroke'
5. *Infections*
   Increased susceptibility to:
   (i) Boils and carbuncles
   (ii) Candidiasis ('thrush'), which may cause vulval itching
   (iii) Tuberculosis
6. *Coma*
   (i) Diabetic ketosis (q.v.)
   (ii) Hypoglycaemia (p. 105)

DIABETIC KETOSIS

This condition is characterized by hyperglycaemia and ketosis. It is a medical emergency which if untreated leads to coma and death.

Clinical features

1. Gradual onset of weakness and drowsiness over several days, often precipitated by infection, injury or lack of insulin
2. Polyuria, polydipsia and dehydration
3. Deep breathing ('air hunger'), with smell of acetone on the breath
4. Anorexia, abdominal pain and vomiting

Treatment

Principles:
1. Treat the precipitating cause e.g. infection
2. Correct the dehydration and restore the electrolyte balance
3. Re-establish the normal blood sugar level
No inflexible rules can be given but most patients in diabetic coma or pre-

coma require 40 to 120 units of soluble insulin (half i.v. and half i.m.) initially, and a saline infusion. Blood is taken immediately for glucose, urea and electrolytes and further treatment depends on the results, with subsequent blood tests at frequent intervals. Hypoglycaemia and hypokalaemia are likely to occur during the recovery stage unless prevented by the infusion of glucose and potassium.

Naso-gastric suction is often required initially.

HYPOGLYCAEMIC COMA

Due to decreased blood glucose (usually below 2.5 mmol/l). Usually precipitated by exercise, a missed meal or insulin overdosage.

Clinical features

1. Rapid onset of anxiety, hunger, headache, irritability or unusual behaviour which may progress to coma within a few minutes
2. Rapid bounding pulse, fine tremor, dilated pupils, pallor and sweating
3. Epilepsy may occur, and severe or recurrent hypoglycaemia can cause irreversible cerebral changes or even death

Treatment

Give glucose immediately, by mouth if the patient will co-operate. Failing that, restrain the patient and the doctor will give 20 ml of 50 per cent dextrose intravenously. Glucagon injection (0.5 to 1 mg subcutaneously) is a suitable alternative.

Management of diabetic patients

Life-long careful control of the diabetes is required to postpone complications. The urine must be tested regularly and kept as sugar-free as possible.

There are two main types:

1. Juvenile diabetes

Thin young patients who need subcutaneous insulin injections at least once daily. Their physical exercise and diet should be as regular as possible to allow good control to be achieved. Such patients must be taught:

  (i) The importance of good control and how to achieve it

  (ii) How and when to test their urine

  (iii) The techniques of subcutaneous injection, sterilization, insulin dosages etc.

  (iv) The estimation of meal portions according to their dietary allowance

  (v) How to recognize and avert hypoglycaemia

  (vi) The importance of personal hygiene to prevent infection

  (vii) The importance of care of the feet to prevent ulcers

Insulin injections

These are three main types:

  (i) Rapidly acting but of short duration (6 to 8 hours) e.g. *Soluble insulin*

(ii) Intermediate e.g. *Insulin zinc suspension* (lente insulin)

(iii) Slow but prolonged action (over 24 hours) e.g. *Protamine zinc insulin*

2. Maturity-onset diabetes

Older obese patients who need to reduce to their ideal weight. They can then be controlled on a low carbohydrate diet (e.g. 150 g daily), with the addition of oral hypoglycaemic drugs if necessary.

All elderly diabetic patients should see a chiropodist regularly to prevent corns, ingrowing toe-nails etc. which can lead to infection, ulceration and gangrene.

Oral hypoglycaemic drugs

(i) *Sulphonylureas*

These act by stimulating the release of insulin from the pancreas e.g. tolbutamide (Rastinon) and chlorpropamide (Diabinese)

(ii) *Biguanides*

These augment the action of insulin e.g. phenformin and metformin

FURTHER READING

Drury M I 1979 Diabetes mellitus. Blackwell Scientific, Oxford
Lee J, Laycock J 1978 Essential endocrinology. Oxford University Press, Oxford
Thomson J A 1976 Introduction to clinical endocrinology. Churchill Livingstone, Edinburgh

9 Haematology

COMPOSITION OF BLOOD

Blood consists of three 'formed elements' suspended in plasma:

1. *Erythrocytes* (red cells), approx. 4 to 6 $\times$ 10^{12}/litre
   (4–6 million/cu mm)
2. *Leucocytes* (white cells), approx. 4 to 10 $\times$ 10^9/litre
   (4–10 thousand/cu mm)
3. *Thrombocytes* (platelets), approx. 150 to 400 $\times$ 10^9/litre
   (150–400 thousand/cu mm)

Haemoglobin, which reversibly binds oxygen, is contained in the red cells. The normal range for Hb concentration is:

Men 13.5–18.0 g/dl (or g/100 ml)
Women 11.5–16.4 g/dl (or g/100 ml)

Plasma is a yellow fluid which contains three groups of plasma proteins:

1. *Albumins,* which by their osmotic activity help to control the passage of water from plasma to tissue fluids
2. *Globulins* which constitute the antibody defences against infection
3. *Fibrinogen* and *prothrombin* which are concerned in blood coagulation (p. 112)

The *total blood volume* of an adult is about 4 litres. Of this, plasma occupies 55 per cent, red and white cells occupy 45 per cent, platelets occupy an insignificant volume

FUNCTIONS OF BLOOD

1. Transport

 (i) *Oxygen* from lungs to tissues, and *carbon dioxide* from tissues to lungs
 (ii) *Products of digestion* from intestines to tissues
 (iii) *Products of metabolism* from tissues to liver and kidney
 (iv) *Hormones* from endocrine organs to tissues

2. Defence against infection

 (i) *Humoral.* The immunoglobulins act as antibodies against infectious microorganisms
 (ii) *Cellular.* The lymphocytes and neutrophils act together to kill bacteria

3. Coagulation

There are at least 13 different *coagulation factors* in the blood which interact in a complex series of reactions to form a blood clot when a vessel wall is damaged (see p. 112).

Red cells

FORMATION OF RED CELLS

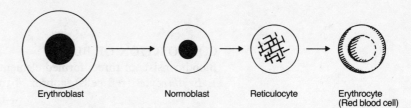

Figure 9.1
Development of red blood cells

Erythroblast   Normoblast   Reticulocyte   Erythrocyte
(Red blood cell)

Red cells are formed in the bone marrow from nucleated precursor cells called *erythroblasts*. The nucleus disappears before the cells enter the circulation. The newly released red cells, which have a blue-staining reticulum, are called *reticulocytes*. Normally less than 1 per cent of an adult's red cells are reticulocytes but the proportion increases with increased bone marrow activity e.g. after haemorrhage or increased haemolysis.

Substances required for the formation and maturation of red cells:

1. *Iron*
2. *Folic acid*
3. *Cyanocobalamin* (vitamin B_{12})
4. *Vitamin C*

These are present in adequate amounts in a normal mixed diet, but deficiency of one or more may occur if:

1. Diet is abnormal e.g. old people living on bread and jam
2. Malabsorption is present e.g. after gastrectomy
3. Requirements increase e.g. during pregnancy

Red cell size

Red cells of the normal size are called *normocytes*.

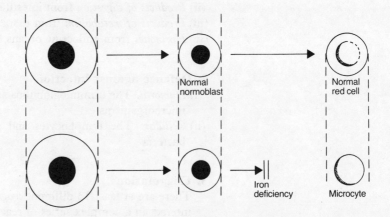

Normal
normoblast

Normal
red cell

Iron
deficiency

Microcyte

Figure 9.2
Iron deficiency anaemia

In iron deficiency the red cells are smaller than normal and are thus called *microcytes*.

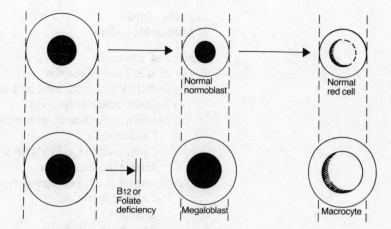

Figure 9.3
Megaloblastic anaemia

In deficiency of folic acid or vitamin B_{12} the normoblasts are larger than normal (*megaloblasts*) and so are the red cells (*macrocytes*).

Anaemia

Anaemia is a reduction in the haemoglobin concentration of the peripheral blood below the normal range (see p. 107). This results in a diminution of the capacity of the blood to transport oxygen to the tissues. When anaemia is present the red cells are usually but not always reduced in number.

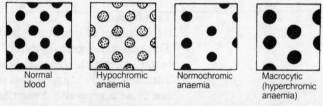

Figure 9.4

In *hypochromic* anaemia the Hb conc. in each red cell is decreased

In *normochromic* anaemia the Hb conc. in each red cell is normal but the total number of cells is decreased

In *hyperchromic* anaemia the red cells are larger than normal, and so they contain a relatively large amount of haemoglobin.

Anaemia may thus be classified into 3 main types:

1. Microcytic, hypochromic (e.g. iron deficiency)
2. Normocytic, normochromic (e.g. acute bleeding)
3. Macrocytic, hyperchromic (e.g. B_{12} deficiency)

Clinical features of anaemia

Symptoms
Tiredness, dyspnoea on exertion, palpitation, giddiness

Signs
1. Pallor of skin, mucosae and conjunctivae

2. Tachycardia
3. Mild ankle oedema

Causes of anaemia
1. *Deficient red cell production*
   (i) Deficiency of iron, folic acid or cyanocobalamin (vitamin B_{12})
   (ii) Aplastic anaemia (p. 111)
   (iii) Marrow replacement with malignant cells
        Leukaemia
        Lymphoma (e.g. Hodgkin's)
        Metastatic carcinoma
   (iv) 'Symptomatic', i.e. secondary to serious illness
        Chronic infection
        Uraemia
        Rheumatoid arthritis
        Primary carcinoma
2. *Loss or destruction of red cells*
   (i) Haemorrhage
   (ii) Increased haemolysis (p. 111)

IRON DEFICIENCY
This produces a microcytic, hypochromic anaemia.

Common causes
1. Dietary deficiency, especially in elderly
2. Bleeding e.g. from intestinal tract
3. Pregnancy

Treatment
Replacement of iron stones by *ferrous sulphate*, 200 mg b.d. with meals. This may cause gastrointestinal symptoms and *ferrous gluconate* may be better tolerated. *Iron dextran injection* (Imferon) may be given intramuscularly if oral iron is ineffective, but it may stain the skin, and can cause a generalized reaction.

FOLIC ACID AND CYANOCOBALAMIN DEFICIENCY
These both produce a macrocytic (also called megaloblastic) anaemia (see p. 109).

Common causes of folate deficiency
1. Poor diet, especially lack of vegetables
2. Malabsorption e.g. coeliac disease
3. Pregnancy
Folate deficiency is treated by giving folic acid tablets.

Common causes of cyanocobalamin deficiency
1. Pernicious anaemia (q.v.)
2. 'Blind-loop' syndrome following gastric surgery (p. 48)

PERNICIOUS ANAEMIA
Cyanocobalamin is absorbed from the terminal ileum, but only in the

presence of *intrinsic* factor secreted by the gastric mucosa. In pernicious anaemia the gastric mucosa becomes atrophic and fails to secrete intrinsic factor.

Clinical features
1. Insidious onset of severe anaemia in middle age
2. Skin has a yellowish tinge, often with glossitis (sore tongue)
3. *'Subacute combined degeneration'*:
   B_{12} deficiency can cause degeneration of the peripheral nerves and the posterior and lateral columns of the spinal cord. This produces numbness and tingling of the feet, weakness of the legs and ataxia (inco-ordination). Occasionally these changes develop before the anaemia.

Treatment of pernicious anaemia
Large doses of B_{12}, followed by life-long maintenance with hydroxocobalamin (Neo-cytamen) injections (1000 μg i.m. every two months).

APLASTIC ANAEMIA
The red cells, white cells and platelets are greatly decreased due to marrow failure. Such patients often die from infection or haemorrhage.

Causes
1. Toxins e.g. benzene
2. Drug reactions e.g. chloramphenicol
3. Many cases are idiopathic

Treatment
1. Isolation from infection
2. Repeated blood transfusion
3. Treatment of infection with antibiotics
4. Steroids to boost the marrow output

HAEMORRHAGE
Anaemia may follow a single massive bleed e.g. from a severed artery, or the repeated loss of small quantities of blood e.g. from peptic ulcer or haemorrhoids. The loss of one pint in an adult produces few symptoms, but the rapid loss of two pints is potentially dangerous. Older people tolerate haemorrhage less well.

Treatment
1. Stop the bleeding if possible
2. Give iron (tablets or injection) or blood transfusion depending on the severity of the bleeding. In an emergency, plasma or i.v. dextran may be infused to maintain the circulation
3. Morphine is useful for restless patients with severe bleeding

HAEMOLYSIS
Excessive breakdown of red cells in the circulation causes anaemia with an increase in serum bilirubin and urinary urobilin. The increased

production of red cells by the marrow produces an increased reticulocyte count in the peripheral blood (reticulocytosis).

Causes

Congenital

1. Congenital abnormality of red cell (e.g. spherocytosis) or Hb molecule (e.g. sickle-cell anaemia)
2. Haemolytic disease of the newborn, due to rhesus antibodies crossing the placenta in an Rh –ve mother with an Rh +ve baby
   Antibody formation is prevented by giving mothers at risk an injection of the same antibody (anti-D gamma globulin) within 48 hours of delivery of the first baby

Acquired

1. Poisons (e.g. lead) or infections (e.g. septicaemia, malaria)
2. Antibody formation, idiopathic or secondary to disease (e.g. lymphatic leukaemia)

Treatment of haemolysis

Varies with the cause. Splenectomy or prednisone may help.

Polycythaemia

Polycythaemia is an increase in the total mass of red cells in the blood. This is estimated by centrifuging the blood to determine the packed cell volume (also called the haematocrit).

Causes of polycythaemia

1. *Hypoxia*
   Inadequate oxygenation of the tissues stimulates the marrow to produce more red cells. This may be due to a variety of causes including:
     (i) lung disease
    (ii) cyanotic heart disease
   (iii) living at high altitude
2. *Polycythaemia vera*
   This is an uncommon disease in which the marrow produces an excess of red cells for no apparent cause. The patients appear plethoric (i.e. their complexion is purple) and they complain of headaches and dizziness. Occasionally the platelets are also produced in excess and some patients develop leukaemia.

Treatment of polycythaemia vera

1. Repeated venesection
2. Radio-active phosphorus or cytotoxic drugs

Blood coagulation

Blood does not normally clot whilst it is in contact with the smooth surface of the vessel walls, but contact with a rough surface, or with certain chemicals released by tissue damage, initiates a complex sequence of events which causes the fibrinogen (a plasma protein) to precipitate out as strands of fibrin, which trap the red and white cells and platelets to form a clot.

Thromboplastin (produced by tissue damage), *platelets* and the other *clotting factors* interact in a complex chain of reactions (the *'coagulation cascade'*) which amplifies the products at each step:

Once a clot has formed, it becomes firmer and contracts over a period of 24 hours or so to bring the edges of the wound together.

Figure 9.5

Tissue damage
↓
'Coagulation cascade'
↓
Prothrombin → Thrombin
↓
Fibrinogen → Fibrin
↓   ←Platelets
Blood clot

Any tendency to clot formation in the blood vessels is counteracted by another complex mechanism which tends to dissolve clot away as it is formed. This is called the *fibrinolytic activity* of the blood. If this mechanism becomes deranged there may be widespread clotting throughout the body (*disseminated intravascular coagulation*). This uses up all the available fibrinogen and this in turn predisposes to a bleeding tendency. Disseminated intravascular coagulation is a rare, but often fatal, complication of many severe illnesses such as septicaemia and major surgery.

BLEEDING DISEASES

Abnormal bleeding may be due to defects in the platelets, the coagulation factors or the vessel walls.

Patients with a bleeding tendency may develop *purpura* in the skin (small reddish-purple spots, also called *petechiae*) or larger bruises (*ecchymoses*), either spontaneously or after minimal trauma.

Causes of abnormal bleeding

1. Platelet deficiency

The platelet count may be decreased (*thrombocytopenia*), or more rarely, the platelets may be present in normal numbers but may not function normally.

Causes

  (i) Idiopathic thrombocytopenic purpura

In this rare condition, abnormal numbers of platelets are destroyed in the spleen. It is treated by splenectomy

 (ii) Aplastic anaemia (p. 111)

(iii) Acute leukaemia (p. 116)

Transfusions of fresh blood or concentrated platelets can be given to control bleeding due to a platelet deficiency.

2. Coagulation defect (deficiency of a clotting factor)

Causes

(i) Congenital e.g. haemophilia (q.v.)

(ii) Acquired e.g. liver disease or anticoagulant drugs

Prothrombin is manufactured in the liver, and liver failure may produce bleeding due to a deficiency of prothrombin. Some anticoagulant drugs e.g. Warfarin, act by preventing prothrombin formation, and overdosage causes a bleeding tendency.

3. Defects of vessel walls

Causes

(i) Septicaemia, especially meningococcal

(ii) Scurvy (Vitamin C deficiency)

(iii) Steroid therapy or Cushing's disease

(iv) Vasculitis e.g. Henoch-Schonlein purpura

Inflammation of the vessels (vasculitis) may occur due to a variety of complicated immunological abnormalities which produce *'immune-complexes'* which lodge in the small blood vessels. The clinical features produced may vary from trivial purpura to life-threatening infarction in several organs.

HAEMOPHILIA

An inherited deficiency of a clotting factor, anti-haemophilic globulin (Factor 8).

The gene for this disorder is always carried on the X chromosome and it is recessive, i.e. it will not manifest itself in the presence of another normal X chromosome. Therefore only males are affected clinically (since they are XY) but females, being XX, can transmit the disease to their sons:

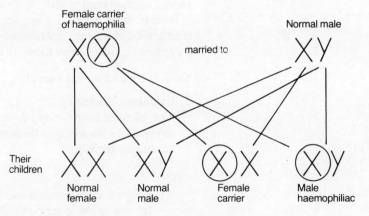

Figure 9.6
X = normal X chromosome
Ⓧ = X chromosome with gene for haemophilia
Y = normal Y chromosome

Clinical features of haemophilia

1. Prolonged bleeding from minor trauma such as tooth extraction
2. Spontaneous bruising
3. Bleeding into the joints may produce crippling deformity

Treatment

1. Surgical procedures must be covered by infusion of fresh blood or Factor 8 (anti-haemophilic globulin)
2. Bleeding into the joints should be controlled by the application of ice-packs, splints to ensure immobility and the administration of Factor 8

Some tests used in suspected abnormal bleeding

1. The *bleeding time* following a small puncture wound in the skin is normally less than 7 minutes
2. The *platelet count* will identify thrombocytopenia
3. The *prothrombin time* is used to identify some coagulation defects and also to monitor the correct dosage of anticoagulant drugs. The patient's blood is sent to the laboratory in a citrated tube (this prevents clotting by removing calcium), and the time taken for the blood to clot after the addition of calcium and thromboplastin to the tube is the prothrombin time
4. The *Hess test* is used to confirm abnormal fragility of the small vessels. A sphygmomanometer cuff is placed on the arm and pumped to around 100 mm mercury for 5 minutes. If the vessels are fragile this increased pressure in the capillaries will produce a crop of purpura

Blood transfusion

Blood groups

There are four main types: A, B, AB and O.

In addition, in Britain about 85 per cent of people have the rhesus factor (Rh positive) whereas the remaining 15 per cent are Rh negative.

Blood for transfusion must be obtained from a donor of the appropriate ABO blood-group and Rh factor. The donor's cells must be cross-matched with the recipient's serum before use, but in dire emergency a patient may be given group O, Rh negative blood without cross-matching.

Complications of blood transfusion

1. Febrile reactions
2. Cardiac failure due to circulatory overload
3. Haemolysis due to blood group incompatibility
4. Thrombophlebitis of the vein
5. Air embolism
6. Transmission of disease from an infected donor (e.g. syphilis, malaria or serum hepatitis)
7. Infected drip site, septicaemia etc. from bacterial contamination of infusion set

White cells

FORMATION OF WHITE CELLS

In a healthy adult about 70 per cent of the circulating white cells are *granulocytes* and 30 per cent are *lymphocytes*.

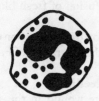

Figure 9.7

Figure 9.8

1. Granulocytes ('polymorphs')

These are formed in the marrow from precursor cells called *myeloblasts*. As the cells mature they acquire granules in their cytoplasm and their nuclei become irregularly lobed. The mature cells released into the circulation are therefore called *polymorphonuclear granulocytes*.

These 'polymorphs' can be subdivided into *neutrophils, eosinophils* and *basophils* according to the staining reactions of their granules. The neutrophils are by far the commonest and they eventually form the *macrophages* which kill and ingest bacteria.

There are also cells called *monocytes* whose origin and function are uncertain.

2. Lymphocytes

These are formed from precursor cells called *lymphoblasts* in the lymphoid tissue (thymus, lymph nodes, marrow and spleen). Lymphocytes are readily distinguished from 'polymorphs' by their dense circular nuclei and scanty cytoplasm.

FUNCTIONS OF WHITE CELLS

The granulocytes and lymphocytes co-operate with each other to defend the body against infection. There are two types of lymphocytes (T and B) which look alike but have different functions. Some of the B lymphocytes turn into *plasma cells* which manufacture *immunoglobulins* (antibodies), and the T lymphocytes cooperate with the 'polymorphs' to kill bacteria.

All types of white cell appear to be involved in producing the changes of inflammation.

LEUCOCYTOSIS

A white cell count exceeding 10×10^9/litre (10 000/cu mm).

Common causes

1. Bacterial infection
2. Haemorrhage or tissue damage (e.g. burns)
3. Leukaemia
4. Malignancy

The differential white cell count

The relative proportions of the various white cells may change in some diseases, and this may be of diagnostic value e.g. lymphocytes increase disproportionately in viral infections, and eosinophils increase in parasitic infestations of the intestine.

The normal differential white cell count is as follows:

Neutrophils	2500 to 7500 $\times 10^6$/litre
Lymphocytes	1500 to 3500 $\times 10^6$/litre
Monocytes	200 to 800 $\times 10^6$/litre
Eosinophils	40 to 440 $\times 10^6$/litre
Basophils	0 to 100 $\times 10^6$/litre

LEUKAEMIA

A neoplastic disorder of the white cell precursors. It is characterized by immature or abnormal white cells in the blood, and there is usually a marked leucocytosis. Anaemia or thrombocytopenia may occur due to crowding out of the red cells or platelets by the white cell precursors, and infection is common, since the immature white cells do not function normally.

There are two main types:

1. **Myeloid leukaemia** — due to proliferation of granulocyte precursors in the marrow
2. **Lymphatic leukaemia** — due to proliferation of lymphocytes in the lymphoid tissues

Both these diseases may be *acute* or *chronic*.

Clinical features of acute leukaemia

1. Fever, malaise, weight loss, anaemia
2. Stomatitis, pharyngitis
3. Susceptibility to infections
4. Bleeding tendency

Acute leukaemia occurs at all ages but is common in young children, and if untreated is rapidly fatal.

Clinical features of chronic leukaemia

The symptoms are milder and more insidious than those of acute leukaemia, and the patients are often elderly.

In chronic *myeloid* leukaemia the liver and spleen may be greatly enlarged.

In chronic *lymphatic* leukaemia the lymph glands are enlarged.

Treatment of leukaemia

This will depend on the age of the patient and the type of leukaemia. In an elderly patient with chronic lymphatic leukaemia causing no symptoms it may not be necessary to give any treatment. In a younger patient with acute leukaemia the following modes of treatment might be considered:

1. Various combinations of steroids, irradiation and cytotoxic drugs such as cyclophosphamide or busulphan
2. Blood transfusions as necessary
3. Antibiotics for bacterial infections

LEUCOPENIA

A white cell count below 4×10^9/litre (4000/cu mm)

Causes

1. Aplastic anaemia
2. Hypersensitivity reaction to a drug e.g. thiouracil
3. Infiltration of the marrow by malignant cells e.g. metastatic cancer. Leukaemia may also rarely present with a leucopenia

Clinical features

1. There is usually a severe sore throat, which may become ulcerated
2. The resistance to infection is impaired, and bacterial infections such as pneumonia and septicaemia are common

Treatment

1. All drugs being taken around the time of the onset of the illness should be stopped, in case the leucopenia is drug-induced
2. In severe cases the patient will need to be protected against pathogenic organisms by isolation in a special cubicle with 'reverse barrier nursing' to prevent transmission of organisms from the staff to the patient
3. Signs of infection must be looked for frequently, and appropriate antibiotics given early in the course of infection

The lymphatic system

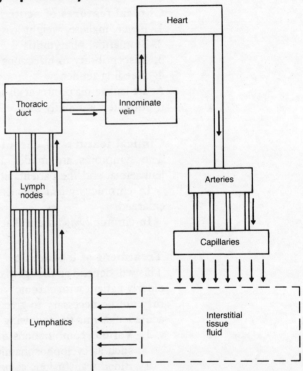

Figure 9.9
The lymphatic circulation

In a healthy person, small volumes of plasma are continually leaking from the capillaries into the small spaces between the tissue cells to form the *interstitial fluid*.

The lymphatic vessels convey this fluid, which is called *lymph*, from the tissues to the lymph nodes, and thence to the thoracic lymphatic ducts which drain into the innominate vein in the chest.

There is thus a continual circulation of the lymph from the peripheral tissues into the venous blood-stream. Blockage of the lymphatic vessels due to external pressure e.g. from a neoplasm, is thus likely to produce *oedema* (an excessive accumulation of tissue fluid) in the affected drainage area.

Causes of oedema

1. Venous obstruction, e.g. cardiac failure
2. Lymphatic obstruction

3. Hypoalbuminaemia (Low serum albumin)
This causes a decrease in the osmotic pressure of the blood, so that fluid leaks more readily from the capillaries into the interstitial fluid. It may be due to:
   (i) Liver disease, since the liver synthesizes albumin
   (ii) Loss of albumin in the urine e.g. nephrotic syndrome (p. 88)
   (iii) Inadequate protein intake (starvation or malabsorption)

Lymph nodes

These occur at intervals along the lymphatic vessels throughout the body, and they play a vital role in helping the body to cope with infection. Pathogenic organisms are conveyed in the lymph to the regional lymph nodes, where the lymphocytes recognize them as 'foreign' and mount a complicated immunological attack which helps to prevent spread of the pathogens to other areas. Cancer cells may also spread in this way to the regional lymph nodes and stimulate an immunological reaction directed against the cancer.

Enlargement of the superficial lymph nodes may readily be felt in the neck, axillae or groins. Important lymph nodes also occur along the abdominal aorta (the *para-aortic nodes*), and around the bifurcation of the trachea and the main bronchi (*the hilar nodes*).

Causes of lymphadenopathy (enlarged lymph nodes)
1. Infections e.g. skin sepsis, infectious mononucleosis (q.v.)
2. Lymphoma e.g. Hodgkin's disease
3. Lymphatic leukaemia
4. Metastatic carcinoma

LYMPHOMAS (RETICULOSES)

A group of diseases of varying degrees of malignancy which arise from the lymphoid tissue of the lymph nodes and spleen (*the reticuloendothelial system*), but which do not produce true leukaemia with abnormal cells in the circulation. Examples of malignant lymphoma include Hodgkin's disease, lymphosarcoma, reticulum-cell sarcoma and myelomatosis.

Hodgkin's disease

Clinical features
1. Usually young adults
2. Insidious onset of fever, malaise, weakness and anaemia
3. Enlargement of one or more groups of lymph glands
4. Progressively downhill course over several years

Treatment
Deep X-ray therapy or cytotoxic drugs e.g. cyclophosphamide.

Lymphosarcoma and reticulum-cell sarcoma

Recent advances in the identification of more cell types in the lymphoid tissues have led to a more complex classification of these diffuse malignant lymphomas, but for the sake of simplicity they may be grouped as *non-Hodgkin's lymphomas*. The clinical features are similar to

Hodgkin's disease, but the prognosis, though often grave, depends on the particular cell-type involved.

Myelomatosis
A neoplastic proliferation of plasma cells in the marrow which produce high concentrations of an abnormal immunoglobulin in the blood. This may be excreted in the urine as Bence-Jones protein. Anaemia, bone fractures and renal failure are common.

Treatment
1. Cytotoxic drugs e.g. melphelan
2. Blood transfusion as necessary

The spleen

Functions
1. Blood cell formation
   (i) In the *fetus* — red cells and white cells
   (ii) In the *adult* — lymphocytes
2. Destruction of 'worn-out' red cells and platelets
3. Part of the reticulo-endothelial defence mechanism against infection
Despite these important functions the spleen is not essential for life, and splenectomy is beneficial for some blood diseases e.g. spherocytosis.

SPLENOMEGALY
The spleen lies to the left of the upper abdomen, protected by the lower ribs. It is not normally palpable, but several diseases cause it to enlarge (*splenomegaly*), and it then protrudes beneath the edge of the rib-cage, especially when pushed down by the diaphragm during deep inspiration.

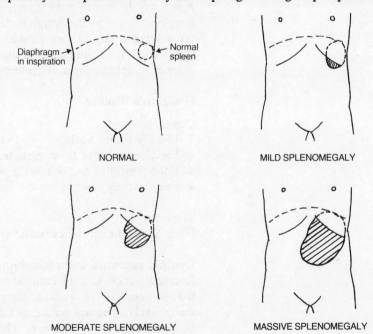

Figure 9.10

Common causes of splenomegaly (enlarged spleen)
1. Infections e.g. infectious mononucleosis
2. Many blood diseases, especially chronic myeloid leukaemia
3. Portal hypertension (p. 60)

Special tests in blood diseases

1. Marrow aspiration
In this technique a needle is passed into the sternum, and a specimen of marrow is drawn into a syringe by suction. Microscopic examination of the cells yields diagnostic information about many blood disorders. A suitable specimen of bone marrow can also be obtained from the iliac crest by *trephine biopsy*.

2. Red cell survival time
In this test a sample of the patient's red cells are withdrawn and 'labelled' with radio-active chromium. They are then re-injected into the patient's circulating blood, and further samples are then withdrawn at regular intervals. The rate of decline of the radio-activity of the blood enables the rate of destruction of the red cells to be calculated. This test is sometimes used to decide whether splenectomy is likely to benefit a patient with haemolysis.

3. Schilling test
This is used to confirm the diagnosis of pernicious anaemia. A measured amount of Vitamin B_{12} 'labelled' with radio-active cobalt is given by mouth, and a large dose of non-radioactive vitamin B_{12} is also given by injection to fill the body stores, so that any absorbed B_{12} is excreted into the urine. The amount of radio-activity in the collected urine then gives an indication of the quantity of B_{12} which has been absorbed from the intestine.

If subnormal amounts of B_{12} are absorbed and excreted, the test is repeated with an oral dose of intrinsic factor to see whether this will correct the abnormality. The addition of intrinsic factor will produce a marked improvement in the result obtained in patients with pernicious anaemia, but it will have no effect in patients with B_{12} deficiency due to other causes of malabsorption (p. 48).

FURTHER READING

Hughes-Jones N C 1979 Lecture notes on haematology, 3rd edn. Blackwell Scientific, Oxford

10 Dermatology

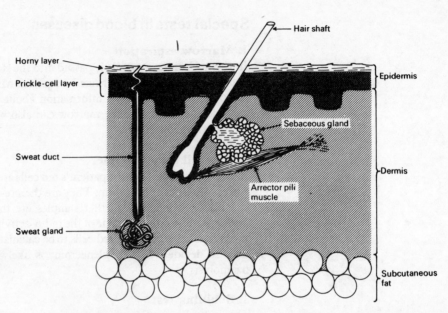

Figure 10.1
Cross-section of normal skin

The dermis consists of a dense mat of interweaving collagen bundles permeated by nerves and blood-vessels (not shown in the diagram for the sake of clarity).

The structure of the skin varies in different parts of the body. Hair follicles and sebaceous glands are absent on the palms for example, but there are profuse sweat glands on the palms, and the keratin (horny layer) is exceptionally thick. Sebaceous glands are prominent however, on the face, scalp and upper chest. In the axillae and perineal regions there are modified sweat glands called *apocrine glands* which secrete a fatty substance which is decomposed by bacteria to form the 'body odour'.

These regional variations in skin structure help to explain the fact that different skin diseases often have a characteristic distribution on the body surface e.g. acne vulgaris occurs where the sebaceous secretion is greatest.

FUNCTIONS OF SKIN
1. Retention of tissue fluids and protection of underlying tissues from mechanical damage and infection
2. Regulation of body temperature
   (i) Vasoconstriction to conserve heat
   (ii) Vasodilation and sweating to lose heat
3. Sensory perception (light touch, pressure, itch, pain, heat and cold)
4. Synthesis of vitamin D (p. 129)
5. Psychosexual functions — smooth skin, attractive hair, blushing

TERMS USED IN DESCRIBING A RASH

Erythema: redness due to increased blood flow through the skin

Macule: an area of discoloured skin (it may be red, blue, brown etc.)

Papule: a small raised lesion. Thus an erythematous maculo-papular rash is composed of small red raised spots

Nodule: a large raised lesion

Vesicle: a small blister (less than 0.5 cm)

Bulla: a large blister (more than 0.5 cm)

Pustule: a blister which contains pus

Weal: a transient red raised area which tends to be pale in the centre as a result of dermal oedema

Scale: easily detached flakes of keratin

Crust: an accumulation of dried exudate (serum) on the skin surface

BACTERIAL INFECTIONS

1. Furuncle (Boil)

A deep abscess of a hair follicle due to *Staphylococcus aureus*. Precipitating factors include diabetes and ill-health, but often boils recur for no apparent reason. Such patients are often Staphylococcal 'carriers' and antiseptic nasal cream (e.g. 'Naseptin') and daily chlorhexidine baths may eradicate the bacteria. A *carbuncle* is a larger abscess which discharges pus through several openings. Carbuncles are treated with incision and a systemic antibiotic (e.g. flucloxacillin).

2. Impetigo

A superficial skin infection due to *Staphylococcus aureus*, sometimes with Streptococci in addition. The crusted lesions, which spread readily, are very contagious. Impetigo is sometimes secondary to scabies or pediculosis. Treatment is with antibiotic ointment (e.g. neomycin and bacitracin) but occasionally systemic antibiotics are required.

3. Erysipelas

A superficial infection due to *Streptococcus pyogenes* which produces a sharply marginated, red, tender, oedematous area, usually with fever and malaise. *Cellulitis* is a deeper Streptococcal infection which involves the subcutaneous tissues, usually as a complication of a wound or ulcer.

Treatment is with intramuscular benzylpenicillin.

VIRAL INFECTIONS

1. Verruca (Common wart)

Usually occurs on the hands, or the soles of the feet (plantar wart), but it can also affect the genital and perianal area. Treatments include salicylic acid ointment, podophyllin, freezing, curettage and cautery.

2. Herpes simplex ('Cold sore')

Recurrent attacks of localized painful erythema with a group of vesicles (small blisters), usually on the lip. Attacks may be precipitated by a febrile illness or sunshine. Treatment is with an antiviral agent called 5IDU (iododeoxyuridine) applied topically.

3. Herpes zoster ('Shingles')

Erythema and grouped vesicles occur in the distribution of a nerve root, due to invasion of a sensory nerve ganglion by the *varicella* (chicken pox) virus. The eruption is often preceded by pain for about two days. Common sites are the chest and face (a branch of the trigeminal nerve).

The rash clears in two to three weeks but severe pain may persist for much longer as *post-herpetic neuralgia*.

FUNGAL INFECTIONS

1. Tinea ('Ringworm')

An irritable red scaly rash which tends to clear centrally. The name varies according to the part affected by the fungus:

Tinea *capitis* — scalp (causes bald patches)
Tinea *corporis* — face, trunk and limbs
Tinea *cruris* — inner thighs and scrotum
Tinea *pedis* — feet ('athletes' foot')
Tinea *unguium* — nails (thickened and discoloured)

Treatment is with fungicidal ointment (e.g. tolnaftate) and if necessary griseofulvin by mouth.

2. Candidiasis ('Thrush')

Due to a yeast (*Candida albicans*) which may occur normally in the bowel, but may infect the skin and oral or vaginal mucosa. It produces red patches on the skin, white patches in the mouth and a discharge from the vagina.

Predisposing factors:

  (i) Moist, warm skin (e.g. body folds in fat females)
 (ii) Wearing dentures
(iii) Diabetes or serious illness
 (iv) Systemic antibiotics or steroids
  (v) Pregnancy and oral contraceptives predispose to vaginal candidiasis

Treatment is with Nystatin ointment, tablets or pessaries. The preparation used varies with the site.

SKIN PARASITES

1. Scabies

A mite (*acarus*) infestation which causes intense itching. This is due to an allergic reaction to the female mite, which burrows into the epidermis.

Treatment is by bathing and then painting the whole body from the neck down with gamma benzene hexachloride (Lorexane) on two successive evenings. Close contacts should also be treated.

2. Lice

Three species (head, body and pubic) can infest man. Their eggs may be seen as small white oval bodies (*nits*) attached to the hair or the seams of clothing.

Treatment is by gamma benzene hexachloride or malathion, and nits are then removed with a fine-toothed metal comb.

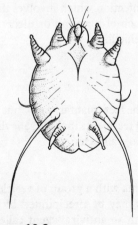

Figure 10.2
Scabies mite

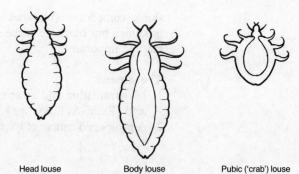

Head louse   Body louse   Pubic ('crab') louse

Figure 10.3

3. Fleas and bed-bugs
These insects bite and cause a small irritable wheal (*papular urticaria*).
Treatment is with malathion powder.

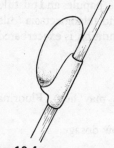

Figure 10.4
Nit

ECZEMA (DERMATITIS)
A distinctive inflammation of the skin in which the prickle cells of the
epidermis become separated by oedema fluid. Clinically there is itching,
erythema, papules, vesicles and a variable degree of scaling and weeping.

Types of eczema
1. *Exogenous* — due to an external cause
    (i) Primary irritant dermatitis e.g. caustics, detergents
    (ii) Allergic contact dermatitis e.g. hypersensitivity to nickel, rubber,
        dyes etc.
2. *Endogenous* — due to an internal or an unknown cause
    (i) Atopic ('infantile eczema')
    (ii) Seborrhoeic dermatitis, usually with a very scaly scalp
    (iii) Varicose eczema of the legs, due to venous stasis

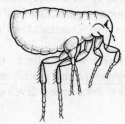

Figure 10.5
Flea

Treatment
If possible the cause is identified and eliminated. Weeping eczema
requires an antiseptic bland lotion such as potassium permanganate.
    Chronic dry eczema requires a steroid or a tar preparation.
    Sedatives and antihistamines may help to prevent scratching.

PSORIASIS
A common inflammatory skin disease with clearly demarcated patches of
red skin covered with thick white scales. The cause is unknown, but the
basic abnormality appears to be an increased rate of epidermal
regeneration in the affected skin. Some patients develop arthritis and nail
changes. Psoriasis is sometimes precipitated by Streptococcal tonsillitis.

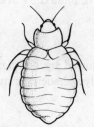

Figure 10.6
Bed-bug

Treatment
1. Topical steroid or tar preparations are useful
2. In severe cases, dithranol in Lassar's paste is used in combination with
   a daily tar bath followed by UV irradiation

ACNE VULGARIS
A common disease of adolescence characterized by seborrhoea (greasy

skin), comedones (blackheads), papules and pustules. The cause is unknown but blockage of the sebaceous duct and infection with bacteria may be important.

Treatment
1. UV irradiation and a variety of topical applications such as retinoic acid (Retin-A) lotion may help
2. A prolonged course of oxytetracycline in low dosage (250 mg daily or b.d.)

ROSACEA
A disease of middle age characterized by redness, papules and pustules of the face, with a tendency to facial flushing and telangiectasia (dilated capillaries). The cause is unknown but the condition is exacerbated by sunlight and heat.

Treatment
1. Topical sulphur or hydrocortisone cream may help. Fluorinated steroids (p. 149) should *not* be used
2. A prolonged course of oxytetracycline in low dosage

URTICARIA
Transient weals with erythema and itching due to histamine release. *Acute* urticaria is often a hypersensitivity reaction to a particular food or drug but the cause of *chronic* urticaria is often obscure. Treatment is with oral antihistamines.

Angio-oedema is a similar process to urticaria which affects the subcutaneous tissues and the mucous membranes of the mouth and throat. Tracheostomy may be needed if laryngeal obstruction develops.

ERYTHEMA NODOSUM
Painful red swellings on the shins which fade to a red-blue colour over two or three weeks. This condition may be precipitated by drugs and infections e.g. TB.

ERYTHRODERMA (*Exfoliative dermatitis*)
Inflammation of virtually the entire skin, followed by desquamation ('peeling'). There is often axillary and inguinal lymphadenopathy, fever and cardiac failure.

Causes
1. Widespread eczema or psoriasis
2. Drug rash

DRUG RASH
Virtually any drug can provoke a rash, and virtually any skin disease can occasionally be mimicked by a drug rash.

Common causes
1. Antibiotics

2. Barbiturates
3. Sulphonamides

Common types
1. Urticaria
2. Morbilliform (blotchy, like measles)

Drug hypersensitivity often causes pyrexia, and if the drug is not stopped renal or hepatic failure may develop.

ANAPHYLACTIC SHOCK

A potentially fatal systemic reaction which may occur if a drug is injected into a sensitized patient. Massive histamine release causes rapid onset of urticaria, angio-oedema, bronchoconstriction and 'shock'. Treatment is with subcutaneous adrenaline and intravenous hydrocortisone and fluid infusion.

LEG ULCERS

Causes
1. Stasis ulcers ('Varicose' ulcers)
2. Ulcers due to arterial occlusion or neuropathy

Stasis ulcers
These are secondary to chronic venous stasis due to varicose veins or previous deep vein thrombosis. They occur above the ankle in middle-aged patients and are often surrounded by varicose eczema and pigmentation.

Factors which delay healing
1. Anaemia
2. Bacterial infection of the ulcer
3. Lack of adequate supportive dressing
4. Sensitization to a topically applied medicament e.g. an antibiotic or lanolin

Treatment of stasis ulcers
1. Elevation of the leg followed by a firm pressure bandage. Initially this is changed daily but later a paste bandage may be applied for a week or more at a time
2. Treatment of anaemia or bacterial infection
3. Skin grafting may speed healing in suitable cases

Special tests in skin diseases

1. Skin biopsy

This is a simple technique in which a small skin specimen is excised for histological examination. This is sometimes combined with a special *immunofluorescent* test which allows various immunological abnormalities to be detected e.g. antibodies directed against the epidermis in pemphigus.

2. Scrapings for mycology

Small flakes of skin are collected and examined microscopically for fungus. They may also be cultured to allow the fungus species to be identified.

3. Patch tests

Substances which are suspected to be causing allergic contact dermatitis (e.g. nickel in jewellery) may be tested by applying them to the unaffected skin under a small patch of adhesive tape. A positive reaction consists of redness and swelling beneath the patch after 48 hours.

FURTHER READING

Burton J L 1979 Essentials of dermatology. Churchill Livingstone, Edinburgh
Wilkinson D S 1969 The nursing and management of skin diseases, 3rd edn. Faber & Faber, London

11 Bones and joints

Bone consists of a collagen *matrix* on which are deposited *calcium salts*. It is continually being formed by cells called *osteoblasts* and removed by other cells called *osteoclasts,* so that changes in the shape of a bone (*'re-modelling'*) are possible according to the stresses and strains imposed on it. When a patient is confined to bed, these stresses decrease and bone tends to be reabsorbed, with consequent loss of calcium in the urine.

RICKETS AND OSTEOMALACIA

Vitamin D (calciferol) increases calcium absorption from the intestine. It is present in milk, butter and eggs and is also formed in the skin by the action of sunlight on a compound derived from cholesterol.

Deficiency of vitamin D causes failure of bone calcification, which is called *rickets* in children and *osteomalacia* in adults.

Causes of vitamin D deficiency
1. Inadequate diet, especially during pregnancy
2. Malabsorption
3. Lack of exposure to sunlight may aggravate a dietary deficiency

Clinical features of rickets
1. Usually an irritable, sweating, flabby infant with a 'pot-belly'. Failure to thrive is common
2. Bone deformities:
   (i) Swelling and tenderness of the ends of long bones
   (ii) Bending of bone may produce bow-legs, scoliosis, pigeon-chest and a narrow pelvis
   (iii) The skull becomes cuboid and soft
3. Dentition is delayed and the teeth decay easily

Clinical features of osteomalacia
1. Tiredness, weakness and bone pains
2. Minor stresses may cause fractures
3. In severe cases muscle weakness causes a waddling gait

Treatment of rickets and osteomalacia
Daily vitamin D with calcium supplements

OSTEOPOROSIS
An atrophy of bone which affects both calcium and the matrix so that the bone becomes less dense.

Causes
1. Old age, possibly related to deficiency of oestrogen or androgen

2. Prolonged immobilization
3. Cushing's disease, or glucocorticoid therapy (e.g. prednisone)

Clinical features
1. May be symptomless, or there may be skeletal pains
2. Loss of height is common, due to vertebral compression, and vertebrae may 'collapse'

Treatment
1. Hormones (androgen, oestrogen or anabolic steroids)
2. Calcium supplements

OSTEITIS DEFORMANS (PAGET'S DISEASE)
A defect in bone re-modelling, with excessive formation of new bone with an abnormal texture. The cause is unknown.

Clinical features
1. Middle-aged or elderly patients with pain in the bone
2. Enlarged skull, kyphosis and the tibiae become thickened and curved anteriorly ('*Sabre-shin*')
3. Increased blood flow through the bones may cause cardiac failure

Treatment
Calcitonin infusions

Joints

There are three basic types:
1. **Fibrous** where no movement is required e.g. skull sutures

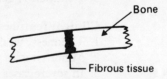

Figure 11.1

2. **Cartilaginous,** where limited movement is required e.g. pubic symphysis

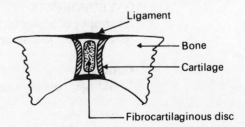

Figure 11.2

3. Synovial, where full movement is required e.g. shoulder, elbow, finger, etc.

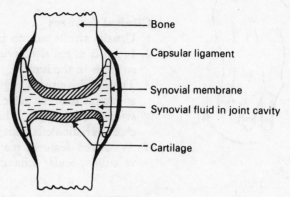

Bone

Capsular ligament

Synovial membrane

Synovial fluid in joint cavity

Cartilage

Figure 11.3

The term *arthropathy* means joint disease. This may be either inflammatory (arthritis) or degenerative.

AUTO-IMMUNE DISEASE AND COLLAGEN-VASCULAR DISEASE

The term auto-immune disease is applied to a group of diseases of unknown aetiology which are characterised by the development of auto-antibodies directed against various tissues in the body. The organ affected is called the *target organ*. Thus in rheumatic fever the streptococcal infection stimulates the production of antibodies which cause inflammation in the joints and the heart, and these are the target organs.

In some diseases the antibodies are directed against one particular target organ, and these are called the *organ-specific* auto-immune diseases. Thus in pernicious anaemia the antibody is directed specifically against the parietal cells in the stomach which produce intrinsic factor, and in hypoadrenalism due to Addison's disease the antibody attacks the adrenal gland.

In other diseases the antibodies are not organ-specific but may affect many tissues throughout the body. In most of these cases there are degenerative changes in the *collagen* in the various connective tissues throughout the body and there is usually some degree of inflammation of the blood-vessels *(vasculitis)*. These diseases are hard to define exactly since their features often overlap, but they may be grouped together as the so-called *collagen-vascular* diseases, as follows:

1. Rheumatoid disease
2. Systemic lupus erythematosus
3. Polyarteritis nodosa
4. Ankylosing spondylitis
5. Dermatomyositis
6. Systemic sclerosis

RHEUMATOID DISEASE

There is no specific diagnostic test for rheumatoid arthritis but in most

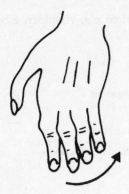

Figure 11.4
Ulnar deviation

cases an abnormal globulin (the *rheumatoid factor*) is present in the blood. This is detected by the Rose-Waaler (latex fixation) test.

Clinical features
1. Usually affects women in middle life (25–50 yr)
2. Presents as malaise, weight loss, sweating, tachycardia and pain and stiffness in the limbs
3. The arthritis usually begins in the small joints of the fingers and wrists and spreads to the ankles, knees and elbows. The joints become hot, swollen and tender. This stage is followed by muscle wasting and characteristic deformities such as *ulnar deviation* of the fingers
4. Associated features may include subcutaneous nodules, anaemia, vasculitis, ocular inflammation and neuropathy

Treatment
1. Rest, with splinting of the joints in the acute stages. Careful attention to posture is necessary and daily physiotherapy is required to avoid joint fixation and muscle wasting
2. Hydrocortisone may be injected directly into the affected joints
3. Systemic drugs:
    (i) Aspirin in large doses
    (ii) Prednisone in small doses
    (iii) Gold injections
    (iv) Azathioprine
    (v) Chloroquine
    (vi) Phenylbutazone or indomethacin
4. Orthopaedic and manipulative measures (wax baths, etc.)

SYSTEMIC LUPUS ERYTHEMATOSUS (SLE)
In this uncommon condition an antibody called the *anti-nuclear factor* is directed against DNA (the genetic protein) in the cell nuclei. The activity of the disease can be monitored to some extent by the level of this DNA-antibody in the blood.

Clinical features
1. Usually young or middle-aged women
2. Fever, weight loss, 'flitting' arthritis
3. Pleurisy, pericarditis
4. Renal failure or nephrotic syndrome
5. Rash, especially in 'butterfly' distribution on the face
6. Anaemia
7. Neuropsychiatric changes

Treatment
Prednisone, azathioprine or chloroquine

POLYARTERITIS NODOSA (PN)
In this rare disease there is inflammation and occlusion of medium-sized arteries and virtually any organ in the body may be involved. Common

features include skin ulcers, neuropathy, renal failure and myocardial and intestinal ischaemia.

ANKYLOSING SPONDYLITIS

Arthritis of the sacro-iliac joints and vertebral joints produces a painful stiff back ('poker back'). The disease usually starts in young men and is progressive.

DERMATOMYOSITIS

Characteristic violet-coloured rash on the eyelids and over the knuckles of the dorsum of the hands, with patchy inflammatory changes in the muscles. Some cases are secondary to internal carcinoma.

SYSTEMIC SCLEROSIS

The skin becomes thick and 'bound down' (scleroderma) with Raynaud's phenomenon and digital ulceration. Systemic changes include pulmonary fibrosis and renal failure.

Raynaud's phenomenon is transient pallor and cyanosis of the digits due to arterial spasm. It is seen in collagen-vascular disease, but can also occur in normal young women.

OSTEOARTHROSIS (OSTEOARTHRITIS)

A degenerative process affecting the cartilage and adjacent bone of a large joint (e.g. hip or knee) as a result of prolonged 'wear and tear'. Usually only one joint is involved but some women have multiple symmetrical arthritis affecting the terminal finger-joints.

Clinical features
1. Pain in the joints, especially after exertion and in damp weather
2. Creaking is heard or felt when the joint is moved
3. May be osteophytes (bony outgrowth) on the dorsum of the terminal finger-joints

Treatment
1. Rest and physiotherapy
2. Aspirin, phenylbutazone or indomethacin
3. In severe cases, orthopaedic measures e.g. walking-calipers, or hip-joint replacement (prosthesis)

GOUT

Recurrent episodes or arthritis due to increased serum uric acid with deposition of urate crystals in the joints. Gout tends to run in families, and it may be precipitated by rich food, alcohol and thiazide diuretics.

Clinical features
1. Usually middle-aged males
2. Sudden excruciating pain in a joint with redness and swelling, accompanied by fever, malaise and irritability. The great toe joint (first metatarso-phalangeal) is classically affected. If untreated the attack lasts for 6 or 7 days

3. Urate crystals are deposited as firm lumps on the subcutaneous tissues, tendons and cartilage (especially on the ears)
4. Renal failure may occur due to uric acid stones and pyelonephritis

Treatment

Acute attack
(i) The affected joint must be carefully protected
(ii) The duration of the attack may be decreased by phenylbutazone, indomethacin or colchicine

Chronic gout
(i) Patients should avoid alcohol and purine-rich foods such as liver, kidneys and sweetbreads (pancreas). Obese patients should lose weight
(ii) Long-term treatment is needed to reduce uric acid in the body, either by decreasing synthesis in the tissues (*Allopurinol*) or by increasing renal excretion (*Probenecid* or *Sulphinpyrazone*)

FIBROSITIS
A vague condition (also called *myalgia* or *non-articular rheumatism*) with localized pain and tenderness in muscles or ligaments. This includes many cases of 'lumbago', painful shoulders and 'stiff neck'. Precipitating causes include exposure to cold, damp and minor trauma.

Treatment
1. Rest and physiotherapy (infra-red radiation and massage)
2. Analgesics such as paracetamol
3. Injection of local anaesthetic or hydrocortisone into the 'trigger-spot'

SCIATICA
Pain in sciatic nerve distribution (back of leg) due to pressure on nerve roots. Often precipitated by coughing, straining, etc.

Causes
1. Intervertebral disc prolapse
2. Lumbar spondylosis (bony outgrowths from the vertebrae)

FURTHER READING

Elliot M 1979 Nursing rheumatic disease. Churchill Livingstone, Edinburgh
Golding D N 1979 Concise management of the common rheumatic disorders. Wright, Bristol
Golding D N 1978 Synopsis of rheumatic diseases, 3rd edn. Wright, Bristol

12 Infectious diseases

Modes of entry

Bacteria and viruses may enter the body in several ways:
1. By *inhalation* into the respiratory tract
2. By *ingestion* and absorption from the gut
3. By direct *inoculation* through the skin

Modes of spread

Infection may be conveyed from one person to another in several ways:
1. *Direct contact* with the patient or particles from the patient (fomites)
2. *Droplets* from speaking, coughing or sneezing
3. *Transmission in food or drink* e.g. water contaminated by sewage, milk from a tuberculous cow, or food contaminated by bacteria from flies
4. *Insects* e.g. malaria is transmitted by the bite of a mosquito
5. *Carriers.* These individuals harbour a particular pathogen but show no signs of the disease themselves e.g. typhoid carriers may remain well but they excrete the organism in their faeces

Signs of a generalized infection

1. **Toxaemia**
   Toxins which are liberated into the circulation may produce fever, headache, sweating, vomiting, aches and pains
2. **Septicaemia**
   In septicaemia, bacteria enter the circulation and multiply. This is a serious condition which causes a high spiking fever and rigors (p. 144). The organisms can be isolated by blood culture, in which blood collected with an aseptic technique is drawn into a sterile syringe, and is then injected into a suitable culture medium
3. **Pyaemia**
   This is a type of septicaemia in which multiple abscesses occur throughout the body
4. **Rash**
   Some infectious fevers are accompanied by a widespread rash. These diseases are sometimes grouped together as the *exanthemata*. One of them, scarlatina is due to the toxin from a bacteria, but the others are due to viral infection.

NURSING
It should be emphasized that good nursing care (oral hygiene, maintenance of fluid intake, suitable diet, prevention of pressure sores, prevention of spread of infection etc.) is of vital importance in the management of patients with infectious diseases.

Viral diseases

INFLUENZA

A common infection due to a variety of strains of influenza virus. The disease occurs in epidemics which spread widely, sometimes over whole continents. It spreads by droplet infection and the severity of the disease depends on the virulence of the strain. In some epidemics it may cause many fatalities.

Clinical features

1. Malaise, fever, mild sore throat, stuffy nose, headache and generalized aches and pains
2. In some cases bronchitis develops, with profuse sputum and cough
3. Depression after recovery is common

Complications

1. Secondary bacterial pneumonia is common. This is dangerous in young children, and in the elderly or debilitated
2. In severe cases, delirium, meningitis, myocarditis and circulatory collapse may occur

Treatment

This is symptomatic.

1. Aspirin is useful for relieving aches and pains and reducing fever
2. Secondary bacterial pneumonia should be treated with the appropriate antibiotic. Physiotherapy will be required in severe cases
3. In very severe cases, intravenous fluid infusion and even injection of steroids may be required

MUMPS

An acute infection due to the mumps virus. The incubation period is relatively long (21 days).

Clinical features

1. Fever and malaise, with pain and stiffness at the angle of the jaw
2. The parotid glands become swollen and tender, and this persists for about 7–10 days

Complications

1. Orchitis (inflammation of the testicles). This is rare in boys, but common in adults. It can cause decreased fertility after the pain and swelling subside

Treatment

This is symptomatic.

1. A semi-solid diet and frequent mouth washes are helpful
2. Systemic steroids are used to hasten the resolution of orchitis. The scrotum is supported, and kept cool, and analgesics are required

MEASLES (Morbilli)

Clinical features

1. The disease starts like a common cold (coryza) with fever, nasal discharge, cough, sneezing, conjunctivitis and photophobia (dislike of bright lights). Koplik's spots, which are pathognomonic for measles, are seen at this stage as small white spots with a red halo. They occur on the buccal mucosa opposite the premolar teeth
2. On the fourth day, a rash appears on the forehead, and spreads down the body as a blotchy maculo-papular erythema
3. The child then begins to improve and the rash subsides over the next week or so, leaving a bran-like desquamation

Complications

1. Bronchopneumonia, often due to secondary bacterial infection
2. Otitis media
3. Encephalitis (inflammation of the brain) is a rare but very serious complication

Treatment

This is symptomatic.

1. Aspirin and nasal decongestants may help in the early stages
2. In babies or debilitated children, penicillin may be used to prevent secondary bacterial infection

Prevention

Vaccination is available and is advisable for weak or debilitated subjects during a severe epidemic.

GERMAN MEASLES (Rubella)

Clinical features

1. The disease starts with malaise, headache and mild sore throat. Swelling of the lymph nodes in the neck and occipital region is usual
2. The rash appears on the second day, and consists of pink macules

Complications

If rubella occurs in early pregnancy, there is a high risk that the fetus will be affected, and the baby may develop a defect such as mental deficiency, cataract, deafness or a cardiac defect.

Treatment

This is symptomatic.

Prevention

It is most important that girls who have never had rubella are vaccinated against it before pregnancy.

CHICKEN POX (Varicella)

Clinical Features

This is usually a mild disease. Pyrexia and slight headache are quickly followed by a characteristic rash. Widespread crops of clear vesicles appear, which after 24 hours progress to pustules. These then crust over to form scabs which fall off about one week later.

Complications
These are rare, but some children develop shallow scars from the lesions. In adults, pneumonia may develop.

Treatment
This is symptomatic, but antibiotics may be required if the spots become secondarily infected.

SMALL POX
This serious and often fatal viral infection was eradicated by a worldwide vaccination campaign, and no cases have been reported since 1979.

INFECTIOUS MONONUCLEOSIS (GLANDULAR FEVER)
An acute infection, usually seen in young adults, due to the Epstein Barr virus.

Clinical features
1. Fever, lassitude, malaise, sore throat
2. Lymphadenopathy and splenomegaly (enlarged spleen)
3. May be a rash
4. Debility and depression which can persist for up to six months

The blood film reveals an excess of lymphocytes, many of which look abnormal. Diagnosis may be confirmed by a Paul-Bunnell agglutination test.

Treatment
None, but prolonged convalescence is often necessary.

Bacterial infections

TONSILLITIS
Inflammation of the tonsils is a feature of many viral diseases, but it is also often due to acute bacterial infection by a haemolytic Streptococcus.

Clinical features of Streptococcal tonsillitis
1. Sudden onset of sore throat, with red swollen tonsils, usually with an exudate. The cervical lymph nodes, especially at the angle of the jaw, are enlarged and tender
2. Associated symptoms are common, including high fever, malaise, headache, nausea, abdominal pain and vomiting

Complications
1. Spread of infection into the surrounding tissues to form an abscess (quinsy)
2. Rheumatic fever or glomerulonephritis, as a hypersensitivity reaction

Treatment of Streptococcal tonsillitis
1. Penicillin orally
2. Antiseptic gargles
3. Aspirin may be given as an analgesic and to reduce the fever

SCARLET FEVER (Scarlatina)
This is an infection by a particular strain of haemolytic Streptococcus which produces a toxin which causes erythema. It usually occurs as a result of direct contact or droplet infection, and the organism usually invades the tonsils.

Clinical features
1. Fever, sore throat, headache and vomiting
2. Generalized erythema of the trunk and face. The area around the mouth is pale and the tongue is first white and furred, and then bright red, with swollen papillae
3. After a week or so, the rash fades and the skin flakes and peels off (desquamates)

Complications
1. Inflammation of the middle ear (otitis media) due to spread of the infection from the throat via the Eustachian tube. This may cause pain, perforation of the ear drum, infection of the mastoid bone or permanent deafness.
2. Glomerulonephritis (p. 88) or rheumatic fever (p. 16) may develop as a hypersensitivity reaction to the Streptococcus.

Treatment
Penicillin is given to eradicate the Streptococci and to reduce the risk of complications.

DIPHTHERIA
This is a serious infection due to the diphtheria bacillus (Corynebacterium diphtheriae). It is now rare in Britain due to widespread immunisation, but it remains a serious problem in some Third World countries. The diagnosis is confirmed by taking a swab of the exudate.

Clinical features
1. Malaise, mild fever, vomiting and mild sore throat, with yellowish-white patches over the tonsils, larynx or nostrils. If the diphtheritic membrane forms over the vocal cords, there may be cough, noisy inspiration and eventual death from suffocation
2. In severe cases there is circulatory collapse

Complications
Toxins from the bacillus may cause inflammation of the heart muscle (myocarditis) or peripheral neuritis. This may affect the pharynx (with associated dysphagia) or the diaphragm (with respiratory paralysis).

Treatment
1. Diphtheria antitoxin and penicillin should be given as soon as the diagnosis is made
2. If laryngeal obstruction develops, suction, intubation or tracheostomy (an incision in the trachea) may be needed
3. In myocarditis, complete bed rest is required

TETANUS
An infection by the Clostridium tetani bacillus, which releases a toxin which affects the central nervous system. The organism lives in soil contaminated by animal faeces, and infection in man is usually due to dirt entering penetrating wounds. All patients with such wounds should receive penicillin and tetanus antitoxoid prophylactically.

Clinical features
1. Stiffness of the jaw muscles (lock-jaw)
2. Generalized stiffness of abdominal and back muscles
3. Painful convulsions
4. Laryngeal spasm may cause difficulty in swallowing, and asphyxia

Treatment
1. Early treatment with intramuscular penicillin and tetanus antitoxin is essential. Tetanus antitoxin can cause a severe reaction (anaphylaxis, p. 127) in patients who have been previously sensitized to it
2. Surgical debridement of dead tissue is advisable
3. Careful nursing and supportive therapy, including muscle relaxants, mechanical ventilation, feeding by nasogastric tube etc

Prevention
Active immunization with tetanus toxoid with booster doses every 5–10 years.

WHOOPING COUGH (Pertussis)
An acute infection of the respiratory tract due to a bacillus, Bordetella pertussis. It is spread by droplet infection, and mainly affects young children.

Clinical features
1. For the first 7–10 days there is only a mild illness, with a dry cough and slight fever
2. Bronchitis then becomes severe, and paroxysms of repeated short coughs occur, terminated by the characteristic whoop on inspiration. During each attack the child becomes cyanosed and coughs up masses of ropy mucus. These bouts of coughing are often followed by retching and vomiting
3. After a further 2–4 weeks the condition gradually settles, but occasional episodes of coughing may recur

Complications
1. Bronchopneumonia with secondary bacterial infection

2. Convulsions
3. Ulceration of the under surface of the tongue, and bleeding from the nose, or under the conjunctiva, may result from the severe coughing
4. The lung damage may predispose to fibrosis, emphysema or bronchiectasis as late sequelae

Treatment

1. The child should be nursed in a warm room, as cold air triggers off paroxysms of coughing. Physiotherapy is helpful in loosening the mucus, and the child must be assisted to sit up and lean forward during coughing bouts. A steam tent may also be useful
2. The antibiotic amoxycillin is effective against the bacillus, and also helps to prevent secondary infection
3. A cough suppressant (e.g. codeine linctus) helps in the later stages when the cough is dry

Prevention

Widespread immunization of the population is advisable. The small individual risk of encephalitis as a complication of the vaccination is outweighed by the risk of serious pulmonary complications or death from whooping cough if the population is not immunized.

In order to reduce the prevalence of epidemic infectious diseases such as polio and whooping cough, it is important that the majority of the population should be immunized. Most infants should be immunized routinely against polio, diphtheria, tetanus, measles and whooping cough.

BRUCELLOSIS (Undulant fever)

A bacterial disease due to Brucella abortus. It is transmitted in milk from infected cows or goats, and since the introduction of pasteurized milk, it has become uncommon in Britain. It causes persistent malaise, gastrointestinal upset, joint pains and intermittent fever. The diagnosis is confirmed by testing the serum for the antibody, and tetracycline is used for treatment.

TYPHOID FEVER

This is a serious bacterial infection caused by Salmonella typhi. The disease is spread by ingestion of food or drink contaminated by the bacillus from infected faeces. The organisms proliferate in the gut and spread via the blood throughout the body. It is more common where water is scarce and sanitation is inadequate.

Clinical features

1. There is an initial influenza-like illness with malaise, anorexia, headache, fever and cough
2. After a week or so, diarrhoea develops with watery green stools
3. There may be petechiae on the trunk (rose spots) and splenomegaly

Complications

1. Intestinal perforation, haemorrhage or cholecystitis
2. Other organs may become inflamed, e.g. arthritis or meningitis

Treatment
1. Chloramphenicol reduces the mortality rate to less than 5 per cent
2. After recovery, serial stool cultures are needed to check that the patient has not become a carrier

PARATYPHOID FEVER
This is a similar but milder disease caused by a different Salmonella.

BACILLARY DYSENTERY
An infection of the colon caused by the Shigella bacillus. The disease is spread by ingestion of food or drink contaminated by the bacillus. It tends to occur in epidemics in overcrowded conditions.

Clinical features
1. Sudden onset of cramping abdominal pain and diarrhoea, with blood and mucus
2. In severe cases there is malaise, vomiting and collapse

Treatment
1. Good nursing is important to ensure adequate hydration and to prevent the spread of infection
2. Oral sulphanomides and antidiarrhoea drugs e.g. codeine

CHOLERA
A serious intestinal infection, due to the Cholera bacillus, which occurs in epidemics in areas where sanitation is poor. It causes violent vomiting, abdominal cramp, and profuse liquid stools containing solid flecks (rice-water). The electrolyte balance must be preserved by infusing large volumes of isotonic saline intravenously. Vaccines can be used prophylactically.

Protozoal diseases

MALARIA
An infection caused by a protozoon, Plasmodium, which is transmitted from person to person by the Anopheles mosquito. It is common in the tropics, and is seen occasionally in Britain in travellers from abroad. The parasites are injected into the blood of the patient in the saliva of the mosquito, and they then multiply in the red cells and are regularly released. Rigors occur at regular intervals of 48 or 72 hours depending on the variety of parasite. Chloroquine is used for the treatment of acute attacks, but in some types of malaria, a second drug such as Primaquine is also required.

Malaria can be prevented by taking a drug such as Proguanil each day while in endemic areas. Drainage of swamps has been successful in eradicating the mosquitoes in some areas.

AMEOBIC DYSENTERY
An infection caused by the protozoon Entamoeba histolytica. This is a disease of tropical and sub-tropical countries. It may cause only mild

abdominal discomfort and diarrhoea, but complications are common, including perforation, stricture and haemorrhage of the colon, and formation of an amoebic abscess in the liver. It responds well to oral metronidazole.

Incubation periods for some common infections

Influenza	2–5 days
Scarlet fever	2–5 days
Whooping cough	10–15 days
Measles	10–15 days
German measles	10–20 days
Chicken pox	10–20 days
Mumps	20–25 days

13 Body temperature

The *temperature-regulating centre* is a group of neurones in the hypothalamus which act as a thermostat.

Normal oral temperature = 36.6 to 37.2°C (98 to 99°F)
Pyrexia = Above 37.2°C
Subnormal temperature = Below 36.6°C
Hypothermia = Below 35°C

The *rectal* temperature exceeds the *oral* temperature by 0.5°C
The *oral* temperature exceeds the *axillary* temperature by 0.5°C
Note that most thermometers take at least two minutes to register body temperature. If hypothermia is suspected (e.g. in a collapsed elderly patient) a special low-reading thermometer is required.

PYREXIA (FEVER)

Common causes

1. *Infection*
   Viral, bacterial or protozoal
2. *Malignancy*
   Carcinoma, leukaemia or lymphoma
3. *Hypersensitivity reaction*
   Hay-fever, drug reaction, 'collagen-vascular' disease (p. 131), etc.
4. *Infarction of tissue*
   Myocardial or pulmonary infarction

Spurious causes of pyrexia include taking a hot drink or a hot bath just prior to the temperature measurement.

Types of fever

Pyrexia may be *continuous* or *intermittent* (for only part of the day). A high intermittent fever suggests undrained suppuration, septicaemia or TB.

A *rigor* is a bout of shivering seen in acute infections due to an increased setting of the hypothalamic 'thermostat'. It has three stages:

1. *Cold.* The patient shivers and feels cold, and the skin vessels are constricted
2. *Hot.* The patient is pyrexial, restless and thirsty, and may have a headache
3. *Sweating.* The patient sweats profusely and the symptoms subside as the temperature falls

14 Drugs

DRUGS USED IN HEART FAILURE

1. Digitalis preparations e.g. digoxin

Actions of digoxin
  (i) Increases the force of ventricular contraction
  (ii) Reduces the heart rate
  (iii) Increases cardiac muscle excitability

Dose of digoxin
0.5 mg three times a day for two or three days to saturate the cardiac tissue; then the dose is reduced to 0.25 mg daily or twice daily. Digoxin is absorbed quickly but excreted very slowly.

Features of digoxin overdosage
  (i) Anorexia, nausea and vomiting
  (ii) Pulse rate below 60/min
  (iii) Extrasystoles, often with 'coupling' of the beats (p. 9)
  (iv) Other arrhythmias e.g. heart block, atrial tachycardia
Elderly patients are especially sensitive to digitalis preparations. The effects are enhanced by potassium depletion.

2. Diuretics
These are used to treat fluid retention due to failure of the heart, liver or kidneys:

  (i) **Thiazides** e.g. hydrochlorothiazide (25 to 100 mg daily) and bendrofluazide (2.5 to 10 mg daily). These increase excretion of potassium, sodium and water, and they also have a hypotensive effect

  (ii) **Frusemide** *(Lasix)*. More powerful than the thiazides. The usual oral dose is 40 to 200 mg daily, but it can also be injected i.v.
  Potassium supplements are necessary with the above diuretics to prevent hypokalaemia. This is usually given orally in a slow-release form such as *Slow-K*, 2 to 6 tabs daily

  (iii) **Spironolactone** *(Aldactone-A)* This antagonizes the action of aldosterone and thus promotes the retention of potassium. It is particularly useful for cirrhosis or the nephrotic syndrome. The dose is 50 to 100 mg a day in divided doses

3. Aminophylline injection (10 ml containing 250 mg)
This may be slowly injected i.v. to relieve the dyspnoea of pulmonary oedema or asthma. Aminophylline suppositories are also available.

DRUGS FOR ARRHYTHMIA
The management of cardiac arrhythmia is complex but the following are commonly used:

1. Lignocaine, procainamide and phenytoin
These suppress ventricular extrasystoles e.g. after myocardial infarction. They may be given i.v. or orally.

2. Beta-blockers e.g. propranolol *(Inderal)* and oxprenolol *(Trasicor)*
These are used for arrhythmia due to digoxin overdose or thyrotoxicosis, and for angina pectoris and hypertension. Side-effects include cardiac failure, bradycardia and bronchoconstriction.

3. Isoprenaline
This is used to increase the heart rate in heart block, and for asthma. It is given sublingually (10 to 20 mg) or as an aerosol inhalation.

ANTICOAGULANTS
1. **Heparin** prevents the activation of prothrombin. It is given intravenously in a dose of 10 000 to 12 500 i.u. and acts immediately. The injections are repeated 6 hrly. to keep the clotting time above 15 mins. The effect can be reversed by **protamine**
2. **Warfarin** prevents the synthesis of prothrombin by antagonizing vitamin K. The initial dose is 30 to 50 mg and the daily maintenance dose is 3 to 10 mg depending on the prothrombin-time estimation. The effect can be reversed by vitamin K_1 i.v.

ANTI-EMETICS
Used for nausea and vomiting.
1. **Cyclizine** *(Marzine)*, 50 mg three times a day
2. **Chlorpromazine** *(Largactil)*, 25 to 50 mg three times a day
3. **Metoclopramide** *(Maxolon)*, 10 mg three times a day

PURGATIVES (LAXATIVES, APERIENTS)
1. **Bran and methylcellulose** provide bulk for increased peristalsis
2. **Liquid paraffin** softens and lubricates the stools
3. **Senna, and phenolphthalein** act by irritating the bowel
Many proprietary remedies exist e.g. *Dulcolax* is useful in pregnancy, and for the elderly

DRUGS TO CONTROL DIARRHOEA
These either increase the viscosity of the gut contents, or delay their passage.
1. **Kaolin and morphine mixture**
2. **Chalk and opium mixture**
3. **Codeine phosphate 30 mg twice daily**

ANALGESICS
The dose depends on the clinical situation e.g. diagnosis, age of patient etc.

1. Aspirin (300 mg tabs)

Chiefly for pain from muscles and joints, but also useful for headaches and dysmenorrhoea. It is anti-inflammatory and anti-pyretic (i.e. reduces fever).

Side-effects

 (i) Indigestion. Prolonged use may cause gastric bleeding

(ii) In some patients aspirin may provoke asthma or urticaria

2. Paracetamol (500 mg tabs)

This does not cause indigestion but overdosage can damage the liver.

3. Codeine phosphate (30 mg tabs)

A relatively weak analgesic which also suppresses cough and produces constipation.

4. Dihydrocodeine *(DF118)* (30 mg tabs)

A useful drug for moderate pain.

5. Pentazocine *(Fortral)* (25 mg tabs or 30 to 60 mg i.m.)

Useful for severe pain but does not produce the mental detachment which morphine does.

6. Pethidine (50 mg tabs or 25 to 100 mg by subcut. or i.m. injection)

Weaker than morphine, but less likely to cause nausea and respiratory depression. Used for labour pains.

7. Morphine (10 to 20 mg by subcut. or i.m. injection)

Powerful analgesic, also produces sedation and mental detachment. Normally given subcutaneously but in circulatory 'shock' i.v. injection is preferable.

Side-effects

  (i) Nausea and vomiting

 (ii) Constipation

(iii) Respiratory depression

(iv) Readily produces dependence and addiction

Morphine is dangerous in patients with head injury or chronic respiratory disease.

8. Diamorphine (heroin) (5 to 10 mg by subcut. or i.m. injection)

More addictive than morphine but causes less nausea and constipation. Useful for terminal cancer.

HYPNOTICS, SEDATIVES AND TRANQUILLIZERS

All these drugs may depress the CNS and their effect is potentiated by alcohol. They also tend to be habit-forming.

Hypnotics

1. **Nitrazepam** *(Mogadon)*

In a dose of 5 mg, its effect lasts about eight hours and the patient wakens fresh. Relatively safe in overdosage

2. **Barbiturates** e.g. sodium amylobarbitone
In the normal dose of 100 to 200 mg they may cause a 'hang-over', and they can interfere with other drugs e.g. anti-coagulants

3. **Chloral hydrate**
Chloral mixture (5 to 20 ml) is useful for elderly patients

Tranquillizers

1. **Chlordiazepoxide** (*Librium*) and **diazepam** (*Valium*)
Both are widely used for anxiety and tension

2. **Barbiturates**
In small doses (e.g. phenobarbitone 50 mg twice daily) they produce sedation

3. **Chlorpromazine** (*Largactil*)
Widely used for schizophrenia, and to potentiate the effect of analgesics in terminal illness

DRUGS FOR INFECTIONS

1. Penicillins

Used chiefly for Gram-positive organisms such as Staphylococci and Streptococci.

(i) **Benzylpenicillin injection** is given i.m. for serious infections which require penicillin, usually 300 mg (500 000 *U*) every 12 hrs

(ii) **Procaine penicillin** has a more prolonged effect

(iii) **Penicillin V (Phenoxymethylpenicillin)** is used orally, usually 250 mg every 6 hrs

(iv) **Flucloxacillin** (*Floxapen*) is unaffected by penicillinase produced by bacteria and is therefore used for 'resistant' staphylococci

(v) **Ampicillin** (*Penbritin*) Not as effective as benzylpenicillin against Streptococci but it has a broader spectrum. Useful for respiratory and urinary tract infections

2. Cephalosporins e.g. cephaloridine (*Ceporin*)

Broad spectrum antibiotics, relatively resistant to penicillinase.

3. Streptomycin (500 mg to 1 g daily by i.m. injection)

Used for tuberculosis but the organisms become resistant unless it is used with a second drug (p. 35). In high dosage it is toxic to the kidney and the auditory nerve. Nurses should avoid contaminating their skin with streptomycin as it readily produces allergic contact dermatitis.

4. Tetracyclines

Broad-spectrum antibiotics (e.g. oxytetracycline) used for chest infections. The usual dose is 250 to 500 mg every 6 hrs.

Side-effects

(i) Gastrointestinal symptoms e.g. diarrhoea

(ii) Predispose to Candidiasis (p. 124)

(iii) Prevent absorption of iron and antacids

(iv) Cause discolouration of teeth during formation in the fetus and young children

5. Sulphonamides e.g. sulphadimidine, up to 6 g daily in divided doses

Useful for urinary tract infections, but allergic reactions with fever and a rash are relatively common.

Co-trimoxazole *(Septrin* 1 tab two to four times a day) is a bactericidal combination of a sulphonamide with a blocker of bacterial folic acid metabolism, which has a broader spectrum than sulphonamides alone.

6. Nitrofurantoin *(Furadantin)* and **Nalidixic acid** *(Negram)*

Both are used for urinary tract infections, especially those due to Gram-negative bacteria.

GLUCOCORTICOIDS ('STEROIDS')

Uses
1. Used systemically in many serious diseases to suppress inflammation and allergic reactions
2. Used in small doses as replacement therapy in hypoadrenalism
3. Used topically to suppress some inflammatory skin diseases e.g. eczema and psoriasis

Commonly used systemic corticosteroids
1. **Hydrocortisone injection** (i.m. or i.v.)
2. **Cortisone** tablets
3. **Prednisone** tablets (5 times as potent as cortisone)
4. **Bethamethasone** tablets (35 times as potent as cortisone)

Side-effects of prolonged 'steroid' therapy
1. *Exaggeration* of the normal actions of steroids
    (i) Hypertension
   (ii) Sodium retention and potassium loss
  (iii) Diabetes mellitus
   (iv) Osteoporosis
    (v) Peptic ulceration
   (vi) Suppression of growth in children
2. *Suppression of tissue reactions*
   This allows infections to spread readily and also 'masks' the clinical signs of infection
3. *Adrenal atrophy* due to suppression of ACTH secretion
   Corticotrophin (ACTH) or its synthetic equivalent, **tetracosactrin** *(Synacthen)* may be injected to stimulate the patient's adrenal glands to secrete hydrocortisone.

Commonly used topical corticosteroids
1. **Hydrocortisone cream or ointment**
2. **Fluorinated corticosteroids**
   e.g. bethamathasone valerate *(Betnovate)*
   fluocinolone acetonide *(Synalar)*

Side-effects
 (i) Prolonged use may cause skin atrophy with striae ('stretch marks')

(ii) If extensive areas are treated enough corticosteroid may be absorbed to give systemic effects

(iii) May cause spread of fungus infection

CYTOTOXIC AND IMMUNOSUPPRESSANT DRUGS

1. **Mercaptopurine**
2. **Azathioprine** (*Imuran*)
3. **Methotrexate**
4. **Cyclophosphamide** (*Endoxana*)
5. **Vincristine** (*Oncovin*)
6. **Busulphan** (*Myleran*)

These interfere with cell division of both normal and malignant tissues. Their effect is greatest on rapidly dividing cells such as cancer cells and the normal bone marrow, gastrointestinal tract, liver and skin. They produce leucopenia, and the dose is regulated according to the blood count.

ELECTROLYTE AND WATER REPLACEMENT

Intravenous infusions are used to replace abnormal losses of body fluids and to correct electrolyte depletion. Special care is required in patients with renal or cardiac disease.

Sodium chloride, 0.9 per cent (normal saline)

This is used to replace salt and water, and the kidneys will then correct any moderate disturbance of acid-base balance.

Dextrose, 5 per cent

This is used to replace water without salt and it will also provide calories.

Sodium bicarbonate, 1.4 per cent

This is used to correct metabolic acidosis e.g. in circulatory 'shock' or after cardiac arrest.

Addition of medication to i.v. fluids

This is required if intermittent injection is dangerous, as with potassium chloride, or if constant blood levels are required, as with heparin.

Latin abbreviations used in prescribing

These are officially frowned upon but nevertheless they continue to be used by many doctors:

a.c.	before meals
ad lib.	as much as desired
alt. die	alternate days
alt. nocte	alternate nights
b.d. *b.i.d.*	Twice daily
c	with
ex. aqua	in water
n. et m.	night and morning
o.m.	every morning

o.n.	every night
p.c.	after meals
p.r.n.	repeat as required
q.i.d.	four times daily
q.s.	a sufficient quantity
rep.	to be repeated
s.o.s.	if necessary (a single dose)
stat.	immediately
t.d.s. } *t.i.d.*	thrice daily

FURTHER READING

Hopkins S J 1979 Drugs and pharmacology for nurses, 7th edn. Churchill Livingstone, Edinburgh

Laurence D R, Bennett P N 1980 Clinical pharmacology, 5th edn. Churchill Livingstone, Edinburgh

Index